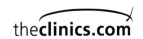

CHILD AND ADOLESCENT PSYCHIATRIC CLINICS OF NORTH AMERICA

Refugee Mental Health

GUEST EDITOR
Schuyler W. Henderson, MD, MPH

CONSULTING EDITOR
Harsh K. Trivedi, MD

July 2008 • Volume 17 • Number 3

SAUNDERS

An Imprint of Elsevier, Inc.
PHILADELPHIA   LONDON   TORONTO   MONTREAL   SYDNEY   TOKYO

W.B. SAUNDERS COMPANY
A Division of Elsevier Inc.

Elsevier Inc. • 1600 John F. Kennedy Boulevard • Suite 1800 • Philadelphia, Pennsylvania 19103-2899

http://www.childpsych.theclinics.com

CHILD AND ADOLESCENT PSYCHIATRIC CLINICS
OF NORTH AMERICA
July 2008
Editor: Sarah E. Barth

Volume 17, Number 3
ISSN 1056-4993
ISBN-13: 978-1-4160-6277-6
ISBN-10: 1-4160-6277-7

Child and Adolescent Psychiatric Clinics of North America (ISSN 1056-4993) is published quarterly by Elsevier Inc., 360 Park Avenue South, New York, NY 10010-1710. Months of issue are January, April, July, and October. Business and Editorial Offices: 1600 John F. Kennedy Boulevard, Suite 1800, Philadelphia, PA 19103-2899. Customer Service Offices: 6277 Sea Harbor Drive, Orlando, FL 32887-4800. Periodicals postage paid at New York, NY and additional mailing offices. Subscription prices are $220.00 per year (US individuals), $344.00 per year (US institutions), $113.00 per year (US students), $250.00 per year (Canadian individuals), $406.00 per year (Canadian institutions), $136.00 per year (Canadian students), $279.00 per year (international individuals), $406.00 per year (international institutions), and $136.00 per year (international students). International air speed delivery is included in all *Clinics* subscription prices. All prices are subject to change without notice. **POSTMASTER:** Send address changes to *Child and Adolescent Psychiatric Clinics of North America*, Elsevier Periodicals Customer Service, 6277 Sea Harbor Drive, Orlando, FL 32887-4800. **Customer Service: 1-800-654-2452 (US). From outside the United States, call 1-407-563-6020. Fax: 1-407-563-8521. E-mail: JournalsCustomerService-usa@elsevier.com.**

Child and Adolescent Psychiatric Clinics of North America is covered in *Index Medicus, ISI, SSCI, Research Alert, Social Search, Current Contents,* and *EMBASE/Excerpta Medica.*

Printed in the United States of America.

CONSULTING EDITOR

HARSH K. TRIVEDI, MD, Director of Adolescent Services and Site Training Director, Bradley Hospital; Assistant Professor of Psychiatry and Human Behavior (Clinical), Brown Medical School; President, Rhode Island Council of Child and Adolescent Psychiatry; Consulting Editor, Child and Adolescent Psychiatric Clinics of North America; East Providence, Rhode Island

CONSULTING EDITOR EMERITUS

ANDRÉS MARTIN, MD, MPH

FOUNDING CONSULTING EDITOR

MELVIN LEWIS, MBBS, FRCPsych, DCH

GUEST EDITOR

SCHUYLER W. HENDERSON, MD, MPH, Postdoctoral Clinical Fellow, Division of Child and Adolescent Psychiatry, Columbia University/NYSPI, New York, New York

CONTRIBUTORS

T. BAUBET, MD, Child Psychiatrist, Department of Child and Adolescent Psychiatry, Avicenne Hospital (Bobigny, France), University Paris 13, Bobigny; Coordinator of the Trauma Center, Coordinator of the Adolescents Division, Consultant, Doctors Without Borders, Paris, France

TERESA S. BETANCOURT, ScD, Harvard University School of Public Health, Boston, Massachusetts

PAUL BOLTON, MBBS, Johns Hopkins Bloomberg School of Public Health, Baltimore, Maryland

NEIL BOOTHBY, PhD, Professor of Clinical Population and Family Health and Director, Program on Forced Migration and Health, Mailman School of Public Health, Columbia University, New York, New York

G. BRODER, MD, Child Psychiatrist and Lecturer, Department of Child and Adolescent Psychiatry, Avicenne Hospital, University Paris 13, Bobigny, France

MELISSA J. BRYMER, PhD, PsyD, Director, Terrorism and Disaster Programs, National Center for Child Traumatic Stress, University of California, Los Angeles, Los Angeles, California

CLAUDIA CATANI, PhD, Department of Psychology, University of Konstanz, Konstanz, Germany

KATHLEEN CLOUGHERTY, MSW, New York State Psychiatric Institute, Columbia University; College of Physicians and Surgeons, Columbia University, New York, New York

JUDITH A. COHEN, MD, Medical Director, Department of Psychiatry, Center for Traumatic Stress in Children & Adolescents, Allegheny General Hospital and Drexel University College of Medicine, Pittsburgh, Pennsylvania

STACY S. DRURY, MD, PhD, Assistant Professor of Psychiatry and Neurology, Department of Psychiatry and Neurology, Tulane University School of Medicine, New Orleans, Louisiana

THOMAS ELBERT, PhD, Department of Psychology, University of Konstanz, Konstanz, Germany

B. HEIDI ELLIS, PhD, Associate Director, Children's Hospital Center for Refugee Trauma, Children's Hospital Boston, Boston, Massachusetts

JASWANT GUZDER, MD, Associate Professor, Department of Psychiatry, McGill University; Director of Child Psychiatry, Sir Mortimer B. Davis Jewish General Hospital, Montreal, Quebec, Canada

CHRISTOPHER M. LAYNE, PhD, Director, Treatment and Intervention Programs, National Center for Child Traumatic Stress, University of California, Los Angeles, Los Angeles, California

ERIC LEWANDOWSKI, MSc, Teachers College, Columbia University, New York, New York

STUART L. LUSTIG, MD, MPH, Assistant Professor, Director of Child Psychiatry Training, Department of Psychiatry, University of California San Francisco, San Francisco, California

ANTHONY MANNARINO, PhD, Professor and Vice President, Department of Psychiatry, Allegheny General Hospital, Drexel University College of Medicine, Pittsburgh, Pennsylvania

M.R. MORO, MD, PhD, Child Psychiatrist, Professor and Head, Department of Child and Adolescent Psychiatry, Avicenne Hospital (Bobigny, France), University Paris 13, Bobigny; Technical Advisor, Doctors Without Borders, Paris, France

LAURA K. MURRAY, PhD, Assistant Professor, Boston University School of Public Health, Center for International Health and Development, Boston, Massachusetts

RICHARD NEUGEBAUER, PhD, New York State Psychiatric Institute, Columbia University; College of Physicians and Surgeons, Columbia University, New York, New York

FRANK NEUNER, PhD, Department of Psychology, University of Konstanz, Konstanz, Germany

LOUISE K. NEWMAN, FRANZCP, PhD, Perinatal and Infant Psychiatry, School of Medicine and Public Health Faculty of Health, The University of Newcastle, Callaghan Campus, University Drive, Callaghan, Newcastle, New South Wales, Australia

GRACE ONYANGO, MA, World Vision Uganda, Kampala, Uganda

ROBERT S. PYNOOS, MD, MPH, Co-Director, National Center for Child Traumatic Stress, University of California, Los Angeles, Los Angeles, California

D. REZZOUG, MD, Child Psychiatrist and Lecturer, Department of Child and Adolescent Psychiatry, Avicenne Hospital, University Paris 13, Bobigny, France; Consultant, Doctors Without Borders

CÉCILE ROUSSEAU, MD, MSc, Associate Professor, Department of Psychiatry, Division of Social and Cultural Psychiatry, Montreal, Quebec, Canada

MARTINA RUF, MA, Department of Psychology, University of Konstanz, Konstanz, Germany

ELISABETH SCHAUER, PhD, Department of Psychology, University of Konstanz, Konstanz, Germany

MAGGIE SCHAUER, PhD, Department of Psychology, University of Konstanz, Konstanz, Germany

MICHAEL S. SCHEERINGA, MD, MPH, Associate Professor of Psychiatry and Neurology, Department of Psychiatry and Neurology, Tulane University School of Medicine, New Orleans, Louisiana

JO SORNBORGER, PsyD, Manager, Terrorism and Disaster Programs, National Center for Child Traumatic Stress, University of California, Los Angeles, Los Angeles, California

LIESBETH SPEELMAN, MA, War Child Holland, Gulu, Uganda

ZACHARY STEEL, MPsychol(Clinical), Centre for Population Mental Health Research, Sydney South West Area Health Service and Psychiatry Research and Teaching Unit School of Psychiatry, University of New South Wales, Sydney, New South Wales, Australia

TRACI R. STEIN, MPH, Teachers College, Columbia University, New York, New York

ALAN M. STEINBERG, PhD, Associate Director, National Center for Child Traumatic Stress, University of California, Los Angeles, Los Angeles, California

O. TAÏEB, MD, PhD, Child Psychiatrist, Department of Child and Adolescent Psychiatry, Avicenne Hospital, University Paris 13, Bobigny, France

LAKSHIKA TENNAKOON, MSc, Department of Psychiatry, University of California San Francisco, San Francisco, California

HELEN VERDELI, PhD, Assistant Professor of Psychology in Education, Columbia University; Adjunct Assistant Professor of Psychology in Psychiatry, New York State Psychiatric Institute, Columbia University; College of Physicians and Surgeons, Columbia University, New York, New York

STEVAN WEINE, MD, Professor of Psychiatry, Department of Psychiatry, College of Medicine, University of Illinois at Chicago, Chicago, Illinois

CHARLES H. ZEANAH, MD, Sellers Polchow Professor, and Vice Chair for Child and Adolescent Psychiatry, Department of Psychiatry and Neurology, Tulane University School of Medicine, New Orleans, Louisiana

Cover artwork Courtesy of Socorro Rivera G., Mexico City, Mexico

CONTRIBUTORS

CONTENTS

This article looks at the experiences of children in war from a psychosocial and social ecologic perspective. In contrast to clinical approaches, it offers a conceptualization of how the impacts of political violence and war are socially mediated. It suggests that psychologic assistance to war-affected children often occurs not through the provision of therapy by outsiders but via support from insiders.

The families of refugee youth in resettlement bear both strains and strengths that impact their children's adjustment and coping. Preventive interventions aimed at helping youth through helping their families should be developed. Given that many refugee youth struggle in school and may have inadequate involvement of their parents, one area in need of preventive intervention is parental involvement in refugee youths' education. The design, implementation, and evaluation of family-focused preventive interventions should be informed by research findings, family resilience theory, a community-based participatory research approach, and a focus on engagement.

Because refugee families tend to underutilize mental health services, schools have a key mediation role in helping refugee children adapt to their host country and may become the main access point to prevention and treatment services for mental health problems. Many obstacles hamper the development of school-based prevention programs. Despite these difficulties, a review of existing school-based prevention programs points to a number of promising initiatives that are described in this article. More interdisciplinary work is needed to develop and evaluate rigorously joint school-based education and mental health initiatives that can respond to the diverse needs of refugee children.

Delivering appropriate care to refugee families requires complex care systems and models that take account of the social, cultural, and political dimensions as well as the psychologic dimension. Children born into these families are exposed to consequences of their own past experiences and also may be subject to the transmission of the traumas experienced by their parents. This exposure can lead to alterations in these children's individual creative resources. Early, tailored care should be provided for these families, so that the transmission of the trauma and its consequences can be managed or ameliorated.

An estimated 80% of the world's war victims are women and children, a significant proportion of whom suffer from social and psychiatric sequelae of traumatic experiences. Various treatments for psychiatric symptoms related to trauma among refugees have been studied. This article summarizes the literature on therapies involving the creation of stories, such as narrative therapy and testimonial therapies, and other storytelling techniques described on the World Wide Web in the absence of an academic literature. At this point, longer and larger studies of the efficacy of all these approaches are warranted.

FORTHCOMING ISSUES

RECENT ISSUES

ELSEVIER
SAUNDERS

Child Adolesc Psychiatric Clin N Am
17 (2008) xiii–xiv

CHILD AND
ADOLESCENT
PSYCHIATRIC CLINICS
OF NORTH AMERICA

Foreword

No place to call home...

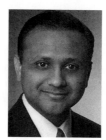

Harsh K. Trivedi, MD
Consulting Editor

As this issue on Refugee Mental Health has come together, I have noticed myself more attuned to my patients as they start talking about home. It is fascinating how much this concept of home—the particular place, the people, the smells, the sounds, and the overall experience—is so vivid in their memory and so vital in their development.

The Geneva Convention of 1951 defined the term "refugee" as a person who because of "a well-founded fear of being persecuted for reasons of race, religion, nationality, membership of a particular social group or political opinion, is outside the country of his nationality and is unable or, owing to such fear, is unwilling to avail himself of the protection of that country; or who, not having a nationality and being outside the country of his former habitual residence as a result of such events, is unable or, owing to such fear, is unwilling to return to it" [1].

So, what happens to a child when political unrest or war rips any notion of home from his or her vocabulary? How does being a refugee affect that child's emotional and physical well-being? How does that child cope with such a schism of experience? What are the short-term and long-term implications of such an event? How does it affect the child, the parents, and the family? What does it mean to lose your home, your community, and all that you have ever known? Where do you even begin to intervene in a therapeutic manner?

I humbly submit that I am ill prepared to even begin answering these questions. That is why I am all the more grateful to Schuyler Henderson

1056-4993/08/$ - see front matter © 2008 Elsevier Inc. All rights reserved.
doi:10.1016/j.chc.2008.04.001   *childpsych.theclinics.com*

for his vision and insight. I also thank the outstanding contributors for sharing their knowledge and expertise. They have created an issue that serves as a primer on the topic and a meaningful review of the current evidence and clinical interventions.

> *This is the true nature of home—it is the place of Peace; the shelter, not only from injury, but from all terror, doubt and division.*
> *—John Ruskin (1819–1900)*

Harsh K. Trivedi, MD
Site Training Director and Director of Adolescent Services
Emma Pendleton Bradley Hospital
Assistant Professor of Psychiatry and Human Behavior
Brown Alpert Medical School
1011 Veterans Memorial Parkway
East Providence, RI 02915, USA

E-mail address: harsh_trivedi@brown.edu

Reference

[1] Geneva Convention of 1951, Article 1A(2). Available at: http://www.unesco.org.

CHILD AND
ADOLESCENT
PSYCHIATRIC CLINICS
OF NORTH AMERICA

ELSEVIER
SAUNDERS

Child Adolesc Psychiatric Clin N Am
17 (2008) xv–xvi

Preface

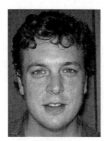

Schuyler W. Henderson, MD, MPH
Guest Editor

The authors in this issue have come together to consider how we can address the suffering and the mental health problems that some refugee children, adolescents, and their families experience as a consequence of displacement. The authors' perspectives may differ slightly, reflecting diverse backgrounds, fields of expertise, and training, but there are nevertheless several common themes. I would like to highlight three.

First, the authors locate mental health treatment in a broader context in which refugees' social, legal, economic, and physical health and survival needs must be addressed. This is not a situation easily reduced to "either/or," nor is it a situation in which it is necessarily beneficial to wait until food, shelter, water, and other basic necessities are available before considering mental health. Certainly, there are finite resources and limited funding sources, but that should encourage us to think about efficiency and collaboration rather than triaged fragmentation of services. We simply cannot ignore how substantially debilitating emotional suffering can be. In any crisis, it is imperative to attend to requirements for living—water, food, clothing, shelter—but the pursuit of these need not exclude attention to mental health. Indeed, mental health must be part of the discussion about these very services. Posttraumatic stress disorders, depression, isolation, substance abuse, irritability, anxiety, pre-existing mental health problems, or emotional suffering affect how people adapt or do not adapt, how they persevere, how they survive, how they connect with the people around them, how they care for their children or meet new peers, how they get a job, learn new languages, attend their child's parent-teacher meeting, and create a new life.

1056-4993/08/$ - see front matter © 2008 Elsevier Inc. All rights reserved.
doi:10.1016/j.chc.2008.03.003

childpsych.theclinics.com

Second, the authors consistently recognize that mental health problems in refugee children and adolescents are rooted in social, cultural, and political environments of displacement and resettlement, as well as the traumas of war, violence, oppression, persecution, and exile. This is about people who have fled persecution, violence, or the threat of violence, and left their homes: their houses, communities, family members, neighbors, pets, schools, doctors, places of worship, places of recreation, cemeteries, and jobs. Many of us have been to talks during which, at the beginning of the presentation, we are invited to write on a piece of paper our favorite things (our photo albums, our computers, our puppies, our very own pillows) and then instructed to tear that piece of paper up, to evoke some symbolic empathy with refugee experiences. In the age of the internet, of globalization, of borders that are at once more porous and more difficult to cross, this simplistic model of loss is not sufficient. Its most useful feature is that it does, briefly, turn the focus on the audience. And so I want to turn the framing of these articles back toward us. The contributions in this issue belong to a scholarly tradition of careful analysis, tentative conclusions, identification of sources, and, when possible, empiric validation. They also belong to another tradition, one that can lay claim to less neutrality and less objectivity. Each article asks what it means to care for people who have had their homes taken from them. This begets another series of questions: whom do we welcome to our shores and why? Several of the authors touch on this in their discussion of the definitions of "refugee," or when they discuss how we conceptualize families or how we detain people at the border. And, after that, what do we expect of refugees in particular and immigrants in general? How much suffering do they experience, how much should they experience, and what should we be doing to alleviate that suffering? Should they be getting jobs? Should they be healthy, productive members of their host country? What sort of parents should they be? What sort of kids should they be? These are questions buried deep within these contributions.

Finally, the authors recognize how incomplete the research is that guides treatment decisions for these very vulnerable, but resilient populations. In this issue, authors consider individuals, parent–child dyads, families, and schools; the authors consider ways of telling stories and how to structure the encounter so that it is healing. But, as each author acknowledges, there is not a lot of evidence. If anything, I would hope that these articles form a backdrop against which we can move forward. The articles are full of questions worth asking and worth answering; I hope that they will inspire people to pursue further investigation.

Schuyler W. Henderson, MD, MPH
Division of Child and Adolescent Psychiatry
Columbia University/NYSPI
Unit 78, 1051 Riverside Drive
New York, NY 10032, USA

E-mail address: hendersss@childpsych.columbia.edu

ELSEVIER
SAUNDERS

Child Adolesc Psychiatric Clin N Am
17 (2008) 497–514

CHILD AND
ADOLESCENT
PSYCHIATRIC CLINICS
OF NORTH AMERICA

Political Violence and Development: An Ecologic Approach to Children in War Zones

Neil Boothby, PhD

Mailman School of Public Health, Columbia University, 60 Haven Avenue B-4, New York, NY 10032, USA

Today's estimates say there are more than 9.9 million refugees living outside their own countries and there are another 25 million internally displaced people (IDP) [1]. At least half of these victims of wars and ethnic conflict are children, many of whom have been exposed directly or indirectly to violence. One study of refugee children who sought asylum in Europe, for example, found that 60% of them had been exposed to violence [2]. Children displaced within war-affected countries may be exposed to violence and additional tragedies in even greater numbers and for longer periods of time. In Rwanda, a 1996 survey found that 96% of children interviewed had witnessed violence, 80% had lost a family member, and 70% had seen someone killed or injured [3].

Children also serve as combatants in today's wars. A recent initiative by human rights advocates identified 36 countries in which children comprise significant percentages of national standing armies, guerrilla groups, or both [4]. The "child soldier," however, is only the most visible manifestation of a much broader concern. Today, children also are caught in the ideological struggles that accompany political and ethnic strife. Different sides teach their own solutions to the ills of a given nation, trying to capture the loyalty and imagination of one generation of girls and boys so that a particular vision of "progress," "justice," or "nationhood" will be imbued into succeeding generations. Guerrilla organizers use highly impoverished circumstances to politicize villages and to recruit boys and girls into their cause. At the same time, governments often force children from these same rural zones into national armies. Youth wings of liberation movements and political parties increasingly are being militarized and used to terrorize civilians in

E-mail address: nb2101@columbia.edu

doi:10.1016/j.chc.2008.02.004
childpsych.theclinics.com

a number of nations as well. The inability to ensure children's neutrality and safety from political strife is a principal cause of refugee flight.

Operational realities

The dangerous circumstances faced by children in war zones point to an urgent need to develop strategies to prevent or ameliorate the negative psychologic and social effects of exposure to political and ethnic violence. The development of psychosocial programs for war-affected children is still in its infancy, however; only a handful of these efforts have been developed as integral components of broader relief efforts and development systems; and very few have been evaluated in ways that demonstrate positive outcomes or impacts [5]. As a result, psychosocial programming remains marginalized from mainstream humanitarian response efforts, with little or no connection to broader assistance and protection operations.

Part of the challenge is that armed conflicts and refugee crises are delimited as situations requiring emergency responses. Emergency responses, in turn, tend to be defined in logistical terms: how many tons of food, tents, medicines, and clothing can be delivered in the shortest period of time [6]. Failure to respond quickly and efficiently to these immediate needs can result in thousands of deaths. Nonmaterial needs are much more difficult to identify and quantify. The logistical and methodologic challenges of identifying, quantifying, and proposing rapid solutions to enable children to cope better with the loss of a parent or to come to terms with the aftermath of witnessing murder simply have not been worked out. Psychosocial responses therefore remain a "phase two" concern—a set of issues that are addressed when the situation "settles down," provided donor funds still are available.

Paradoxically, the fact that war-related trauma is widespread among civilian populations also works against serious commitments to mental health assistance. At a time when donor agencies are asking major international organizations to economize—to assist more war and refugee victims with fewer resources—the trauma statistics seem to be overwhelming. Instead of identifying a significant but containable problem with clear solutions, the numbers (eg, 95% of one war-affected population was found to be suffering from posttraumatic stress disorder [PTSD] [7]) point to a problem that affects vast numbers of people but has no clear-cut remedies. From a policy perspective, increasing the funds for mental health programs at a time when food and other material resources are critically scarce may not be perceived by donor agencies or key operational agencies as an appropriate allocation of resources.

Even when funds have been available to address these complex concerns, clinic-based approaches largely have proved to be too narrow and too expensive to respond effectively to large numbers of war-affected people [8]. In recent years, clinic-based programs have managed to treat only an average of 200 war-affected individuals per year, but the cost of these programs is

10 times higher than that of life-sustaining supplies for food, shelter, and basic medical care. Clinic-based programs have not provided a viable, cost-effective model for mental health assistance in situations where tens of thousands of men, women, and children have suffered from political or ethnic violence.

Moreover, concepts of mental health vary across cultures. Western psychology has focused on mental illness and concepts of trauma and PTSD. Although the concept of PTSD has been validated and has value in many developed-country contexts, a focus on trauma can marginalize other effects of war such as mistrust, hopelessness, social exclusion, and the current stress and deprivations of daily life. The diagnosis of PTSD, a product of Western psychiatry and psychology, does not fit well into local concepts of mental health and well-being in many developing countries [9–13].

In Mozambique, for example, many war-affected children had problems sleeping at night because they heard the voices of their dead parents asking why proper burials rituals were not performed for them. Seen from a Western trauma model, these children were experiencing intrusive thoughts and sleep disturbances reflective of PTSD and stemming their parents being killed. Seen from the local cosmology, their parents' spirits were unable to transition to the next world without burial ritual—a situation that was believed to be problematic both for these children and for their community as well. Culturally constructed meanings mediate one's response to potentially traumatic events, making it important to understand local beliefs and to avoid imposing preconceptions about trauma when working with culturally diverse populations [8,14]. A 16-year life-outcome study of former Mozambican child soldiers found that systems of local healing practices (including burial and cleansing rituals) were linked to positive adult outcomes [15].

In the final analysis, both the individual and the society are hurt by failures to integrate psychosocial assistance effectively into mainstream relief and development systems. The physical, mental health, and social needs of war-affected populations are, of course, intertwined. On the one hand, basic assistance is crucial to psychosocial well-being: families that do not have food or shelter or security, for instance, will not be able to care for their children adequately. Economic redevelopment, increased livelihood opportunities, housing, and education are services that also benefit the social and mental health of entire populations. On the other hand, the affective state and motivation level of any given population is a fundamental underpinning of social and economic progress. Children who have been emotionally injured by political or ethnic violence may not be able to concentrate in school, and youth may be unable to take hold of livelihood opportunities when their minds are preoccupied with the past.

The traumatic impact of political violence

Exposure to political violence is associated with an increased risk of both acute and chronic posttraumatic stress reaction [16–21]. Most commonly,

symptoms of traumatic stress among refugees have been assessed using the
diagnostic criteria of PTSD. Although the cross-cultural validity of the
PTSD construct and its appropriateness in situations of ongoing warfare
are sources of ongoing controversy (as noted previously), the constellation
of symptoms that comprise the PTSD syndrome has been documented in
numerous studies of refugees representing diverse national and ethnic backgrounds. Prevalence levels of PTSD among these diverse groups have been
strikingly high, ranging from 40% to 90% [21,22].

Studies of refugee children have revealed a greater variation in levels of
PTSD than seen in studies of adult refugees. Critical factors seem to be
the degree to which children were exposed to acts of violence before becoming displaced [23,24] and the degree to which children were supported during
and after displacement [24–26]. A study of Palestinian children in the Gaza
Strip, for example, found a positive relationship between the number of
traumatic events children had experienced and the severity of the PTSD
symptoms [27]. Forty-one percent of the children met diagnostic criteria
for PTSD at the time of the initial assessment. The traumatic nature of
war-related violence also was examined in a study of Bosnian children in
the beleaguered city of Mostar in Bosnia [23,28]. The estimated prevalence
of PTSD was 52%. Other studies of war-affected children have found lower
rates of psychologic trauma, generally reflecting comparatively lower rates
of exposure to political violence. Miller, for example, found little evidence
of post-traumatic stress symptoms in his study of Guatemalan children
living in refugee camps in southern Mexico (K. Miller, unpublished data,
1994). He attributed the absence of trauma primarily to the fact that most
of the children had spent their childhoods in the relative safety of the camps
and thus had not witnessed the political violence that caused their families to
flee into Mexico 10 years earlier. In contrast to the children, their mothers
experienced persistent symptoms of trauma that reflected the violence they
had experienced directly. The intergenerational impact of this maternal
trauma was suggested by a significant inverse relationship between girls'
mental health and the level of distress reported by their mothers. The relationship was not found for boys, who generally spent much more time than
girls outside the camp home, working with their fathers, gathering firewood,
attending school, or playing with other boys.

Although available evidence suggests a clear relationship between exposure to violence and the onset of traumatic symptoms, the observation
that many children exposed to violence do not develop enduring psychologic
trauma indicates the presence of protective factors that may buffer the effects of potentially harmful experiences. The few studies that have examined
variables that seem to mediate or moderate the impact of violence have
yielded findings consistent with those of research on other forms of traumatic stress. Variables such as the nature of the violent events to which children are exposed, the availability of familial and social supports during and
following exposure to violence, the meaning that survivors of violence make

of their experiences, and the range of coping strategies and resources available to victims of violence all seem to play roles in determining the long-term impact of violence on children's development [25,26,29–32]. For children in war zones, gender and age are significant determinants of the type of violent and abusive experiences to which they are likely to be exposed. Teen-aged boys, for instance, often are at risk of being recruited into fighting forces or detained for suspicion of guerrilla activity; teenaged girls may be forced into fighting forces or suffer sexual exploitation and abuse [14,26]. Several researchers also have found that a critical factor mediating the impact of violence on children (particularly infants and young children) is the extent to which acts of violence result in the loss or psychologic incapacitation of their parents or main caretakers [32–35].

Because war zones present multiple risks to children, their situation can-not be understood in terms of single traumatic events, such as exposure to violence, displacement, a physical injury, or the death of a parent. As a re-sult, a number of researchers have employed a risk-accumulation model [36] to provide insights into the fate of children in conflict and postconflict situ-ations [25,32,37]. This model suggests that most children can cope with low levels of risk, but the accumulation of risk jeopardizes development, espe-cially when no compensatory forces are at work. Specifically, children seem to be able to cope with one or two major risk factors in their lives, but when risk accumulates with the addition of a third, fourth, and fifth fac-tor, there is a significant increase in developmental damage [25]. This model highlights the importance of context in understanding the differences ob-served among children growing up in war zones and in refugee camps.

An ecologic approach

Healthy child development occurs within nested systems of family, com-munity, and society [38,39]. The family, including extended family in many parts of the world, is the key microsystem within which children develop and where basic protections and needs are provided. Outside the family, schools and houses of religious activities provide the first encounter with social in-stitutions and are important spheres of interaction between children, their peers, and significant adults, such as teachers. At a wider, macrosystemic level, children's socialization and development occur within social systems that include norms with respect to children's rights, rules of law, forms of conflict resolution, cultural bereavement processes, and educational opportunities.

Within an ecologic framework, armed conflict is conceptualized best as producing neither masses of traumatized individuals nor a traumatized pop-ulation [40,41]. Rather, an interactive framework that emphasizes commu-nity stabilization, the reduction of risks, and the strengthening of resilience is more appropriate for understanding and developing interven-tions to address the repercussions of conflict. In particular, armed conflict provides an ecologic shock or destabilization that creates a culture of violence that damages child protection and support at multiple, interacting levels. At the level of the macrosystem, internal war shatters societal peace and social trust, contests the legitimacy of institutions and government-defined laws, amplifies poverty and structural violence, and damages infrastructure and institutions of child support, such as schools and health clinics [3]. It also establishes a societal norm of violence, divides the population, and creates structural violence through denial of access to services for meeting basic human needs.

An ecologic approach to understanding children and war thus begins with a thorough examination of the protective capacities (and deficits) of key people and systems that surround them. It should form the basis for thinking with appropriate breadth of potential influences on children's well-being but also should be sufficiently focused to frame clear actions that will promote child protection and well-being. The goal is to identify features of both micro- and macrosystems that together can be seen to form a potential protective shield around children, not eliminating risks and vulnerabilities but protecting children from their full impact.

Historically, parents' abilities to protect their children have been compromised seriously by conflicts, famines, and natural disasters. Crisis-affected families often are in a weaker position to provide material support for their children and also may be too overburdened with survival concerns to provide adequate emotional support. Forced migration and economic pressures often require women to assume work roles that involve longer separations as caregivers from their children than are normal. The stress on families is exacerbated by the collapse of traditional livelihood strategies, which may involve food collection, seasonal migration, and raising livestock, for example.

The protective capacities of other important people are likely to have been undermined also. Traditional leaders no longer may be able or willing to negotiate cessations of military action; religious leaders may encourage violence rather than tolerance; health care facilities may not represent a consistently protective space for children; and schools may become indoctrination vehicles or even recruitment grounds for political factions.

Thus an assessment of the protective capacities of important people and institutions around children is essential. Assessments may need to focus on how the emergency has affected

- Family livelihoods
- Gender, labor, and child-care roles
- Teachers' roles, corporal punishment, indoctrination, and recruitment in schools
- Roles of traditional and religious leaders and their commitments to child protection

Family, kinship, tribal, and, at times, feudal relationships are part of complex socioeconomic systems that maintain order and assign roles and responsibilities to all members of society. Of particular interest from an eco-logic perspective are the expectations regarding children and the features of community life that may be considered protective (or harmful) of them. For instance, a strong commitment to family is an important feature of potential security and stability for children. The widespread practice of informal adoption of orphaned or separated children usually is a key indication of the strength of kinship obligation to protect and care for children and should be part of an early situational assessment. Family stability also is linked with a strong sense of the need for moral education and a clear con-cern that children be provided with clear moral precepts and examples. There also is a range of social and religious customs—from alms giving, to youth groups, to traditional conflict resolution procedures—that are po-tentially protective as well. Expectations and obligations of protecting one's kin—widely cited as a frequent occurrence in context of emergencies—point to social bonds that serve protective functions.

An ecologic approach needs to ascertain the extent to which a given emergency has disrupted the capacity of communities to use fully a wide range of intricate social mechanisms that previously were used to maintain social cohesion within and between villages. Accordingly, it usually will make sense to consider means of supporting or, where they have failed com-pletely, re-establishing traditional mechanisms that have a protective value. There are likely to be other features of community life that—shaped by the harsh physical and economic conditions and deeply engrained cultural atti-tudes and practices —seem profoundly hostile to the welfare of children. Two major concerns that require careful assessment and response in emer-gencies are the commoditization of children as a source of labor and the control of girls (and their sexuality) through marked gender disparity.

The commoditization of children as economic units may be exacerbated by war, famine, and confinement in IDP and refugee camps. Children—especially girls—may be required to remain home for longer periods of time to care for younger siblings. Females also may be expected to assume dangerous roles (eg, firewood collection in hostile environments outside subsidized camps) because such duties would be even more threatening to males. Although emergencies may challenge household livelihoods severely, longstanding cultural norms and values regarding childhood—and especi-ally children's roles in the household economy and gender expectations—will need to be addressed strategically in emergency settings as well.

A similar analysis is required of gender disparity and the subjugation of women. The role of girls in the household economy is a special concern, as is their engagement in the broader labor market. Access to education, infor-mal education opportunities, and other potentially protective activities should be assessed routinely. Female circumcision, early marriage, tolera-tion of domestic abuse, and marginalization of women from decision mak-ing all point to the engrained nature of attitudes maintaining the vulnerability of women and girls. When these and other harmful practices are widespread, decisions must be made whether and how to address these longstanding, socially sanctioned patterns without alienating significant segments of the community.

Community members will discuss some child welfare concerns more openly than others. One must not assume that the problem does not exist because people say it does not. Communities may show a willingness to discuss conflict-related rape or child soldiers, for instance, but discussion of domestic violence and child labor within their own households and communities remains taboo. At the same time, armed conflict often prompts people to look critically at their previous attitudes and practices. In Pakistan, for example, open dialogue with traditional Afghan leaders about their desire to continue to have women and girls treated by female doctors led to the establishment of home-based schools for refugee girls—institutions which subsequently were evaluated as superior learning environments compared with "formal" schools established in camps [42]. Much of what was learned about supporting girls' education in Pakistan continues to be applied in return communities in Afghanistan. Participatory assessment methods in northern Uganda enabled displaced women to discuss domestic violence and rape in a manner that resulted in the establishment of prevalence rates and women's ranking of these concerns as their top protection-assistance priorities [43]. Good practice also is emerging on how to engage children in analyses of their own concerns about protection and well-being [5]. Protection mapping, free-listing, and other participatory exercises provide opportunities for children to identify and rank the risks they face, to identify and rank the actions they and others may take to protect them from these risks, to define what "doing well" means to them, and to outline a concrete plan to achieve "well-being."

Access to education provides protection. Or does it? This advocacy refrain is true only when schools are physically safe and emotionally healing environments. During armed conflict and in refugee and IDP camps, adverse teacher/student ratios often soar to even higher levels; already harsh disciplinary practices deteriorate into public humiliation and corporal punishment, peer teasing may worsen into overt bullying, and boys and girls may be at greater risk for sexual exploitation than ever before. Ensuring that these core protective ingredients are in place is a key child welfare concern. Core protective factors in schools include adequate teacher/student ratios; elimination of humiliation, bullying and corporal punishment; and safeguards against sexual abuse and exploitation. A review of education in emergencies suggests that school enrollment rates do not always drop in an emergency; sometimes they actually increase [44]. Key factors include

- History of enrollment before the emergency
- Short-term economic survival needs
- Safety and distance to schools

- Presence or absence of funding for emergency education
- Fees levied by teachers and/or school committees

Particular attention needs to be paid to the educational needs of vulnerable groups, including, among others, children in female-headed households; households in which grandparents or older siblings are the primary caregivers; and teenage females with babies of their own. Emotional, social, and material supports often are required to enable these groups of children to realize their right to education in emergency settings.

In addition to schools, children's clubs, recreation programs, and youth committees have the potential to provide protective environments for children and also expose them to activities that promote self-esteem, choice, autonomy, and other factors that have been linked to resilience in childhood [25,45]. A key factor in determining whether such community mechanisms are capable of fostering self-confidence and children's engagement in community affairs is the attitudes and behaviors of the people who run them. Several evaluations have noted that an authoritarian, teacher-oriented approach to decision making is not conducive to child participation in important community affairs [46].

Finally, considerable evidence suggests that curriculum becomes highly politicized in situations of armed conflict and that schools often serve as recruitment grounds for one or both opposing factions [26]. Youth, in particular, may engage actively in the political discourse regarding the current crisis and have strong feelings about what has happened to their communities and what lies ahead. Although such participation may be valuable and broadly welcomed, during an emergency particular attention needs to be paid to the political manipulation of children in schools, religious institutions, youth groups, and other social networks.

Clearly children's welfare is affected significantly by the attitudes and actions of all parties engaged in the conflict. There are enormous challenges to protection when government authorities or other parties to a conflict instigate or refuse to prevent human rights violations. Intentional human rights abuse requires protective activities aimed at government and/or other responsible actors. Key modes of protection action may include denunciation (pressing authorities through public discourse into meeting their obligations) to accomplish policy change objectives, for example, and substitution (directly providing services to victims of violations) to accomplish assistance and support needs. In contrast, if authorities are not engaged directly in rights violations, protection actions may include persuasion (convincing authorities through private dialogue) or mobilization (engaging leaders, political bodies, or states that have the capacity to influence authorities to satisfy their obligations) and empowering national or local structures to carry out their functions to protect and assist affected populations.

Government commitment to respecting, protecting, and fulfilling child rights and welfare concerns protection is essential. Often governments deny that there is a problem in their own country, when in reality exploitation of children is found all around the world. In such situations, pressure on the government is required from both "inside" and "outside" actors to create stronger legal frameworks that comply with international legal standards, policies, and programs and to enforce and implement them to protect children.

In situations of armed conflict, efforts to obtain commitments from authorities to fulfilling child protection rights often must be extended both to the government and to other duty barriers as well. These include other parties to the conflict and armed groups that influence or control populations in remote areas of the country or in refugee or IDP camps. Even if acknowledgment of and negotiations with other political/military actors is difficult or forbidden, obtaining the commitment of all duty barriers to adhere to child rights standards is an important objective.

Finally, international agencies may assume roles in emergencies that place them in positions of serving as de facto or on-the-ground authorities (eg, when peacekeeping missions are undertaken and when United Nation or nongovernmental organizations assume lead management roles or engage in direct delivery of services in refugee or IDP camps). Their commitment and capacity to protect child welfare and rights concerns must be assessed and developed as well.

Core psychosocial programs

As noted previouisly, political violence may produce extensive damage and loss of social and economic supports. Parents, family, and friends may be killed or wounded. In diverse war zones around the world, parents, overwhelmed by their war experiences and by day-to-day-realities, may lapse into ineffective parenting or may be in a poor position to make good decisions about their children's well-being [47]. Displacement may tear children away from friends and rob them of support from a favorite teacher or extended family member. War exacerbates poverty, increases economic stresses on families, and robs people of productive employment, farming, and social roles. Governments and other parties to a conflict may attack segments of civilian populations, rob them of their farms and livestock, and deny them access to health and other essential services.

In this context, a clinical mental health focus is too narrow and individualistic to provide an appropriate point of entry for intervention work [8,26,48]. A stronger approach is to focus on mobilizing communities to strengthen basic care and support for children [47,49,50]. Research suggests that collective engagement around meeting children's needs helps re-establish a collective focus, build cooperation, and increase hope among community members. As communities take steps to care for their children, they regain the sense of control that traumatic experiences undermine, and their sense of self-reliance provides a platform for longer-term development and movement beyond a reactive crisis mode [47,51]. The following discussion outlines three core psychosocial programs that have proven to be essential for children in war zones.

Protecting separated children

In various conflicts the number of children separated from their families has ranged from a few hundred to several hundreds of thousands [33,52]. Although the number of separated children is historically underestimated, it is widely accepted that separated children are among the groups of children most at risk in war and refugee crises. Effective programming for separated children in emergencies includes activities designed to prevent separation and, when unsuccessful, to provide interim care and reunite children with separated loved ones as rapidly as possible [33,53–55].

In general, the separation of children from their families can be grouped into two primary categories: involuntary and voluntary [33]. The distinction between these two groups is useful because it provides important insights into the intent of the parent/child separation, the possibility of preventing such separations in the future, and whether reunion is desirable or even possible. Involuntary separation indicates that the separation has taken place against the will of the parents. These separations include situations in which children are abducted or physically taken from the parents against their will, are lost or separated accidentally from their parents, are orphaned or living in a new care situation because both parents are deceased, intentionally leave their parents without parental consent (runaways), or are removed from their parents as a result of the loss or separation of parental rights.

In contrast, voluntary separations occur with the parents' consent. These separations include situations in which children are abandoned or deserted by parents who have no intention of reunion, are entrusted or voluntarily placed in the care of another adult or in an institution by parents who intend to reclaim them, are surrendered by parents who have given up parental rights permanently, or are independent and living apart from their parents with parental consent. Given the variable nature of separation—and the implications for future actions—it is critical to assess each child's separation experience individually and as accurately as possible.

Prevention of child–family separations is a key focus of emergency responses. Voluntary abandonment can be lessened, for example, by ensuring that distribution systems are equitable and that food and water and medical, educational, and social services are available for all families. Voluntary separations have increased significantly when relief efforts established preferential food, education, and resettlement opportunities for children who are alone versus those who remained with families. Specific efforts should be made to support children in their own communities and to identify particularly vulnerable families, such as single-parent or child-headed households.

Interim care in conflict settings should be culturally appropriate, should encourage age-appropriate development, and should allow siblings to stay together. Available evidence suggests that foster family care provides younger children from varied cultural contexts essential attachment opportunities and that even severely distressed school age and younger children adapt reasonably well psychologically and physically to foster settings [33,56,57]. Peer-group care has been found to be effective in meeting the developmental needs of adolescents in times of family separation and armed conflict. In many cases, peer-group care consists of a small number of teenagers living together under the supervision of one or two adults who act as parental figures [55]. In the absence of positive adult role models, however, disciplinary problems, poor coping strategies, and limited academic performance have been noted. International adoption of war-affected and refugee children is rarely an appropriate interim care response [33,54].

Tracing and reunification efforts should be initiated within a short period of time. Although approaches to tracing differ according to the context of the emergency, the majority of comprehensive tracing efforts contain the following elements [54]:

- Identification: the process of establishing which children have been separated from their families or other caretakers and where they may be found
- Registration: the compilation of key personal data: full name, date and place of birth, father's and mother's names, former address, and present location (This information is collected for the purpose of establishing the identity of the child, for protection, and to facilitate tracing.)
- Documentation: the process of recording further information to meet the specific needs of the child, including tracing, and to make plans for the child's future (Documentation is a part of an ongoing registration process.)
- Tracing: the process of searching for family members or primary legal or customary caregivers (The term also refers to the search for children by parents. The objective is reunification of children with parents or other close relatives.)
- Reunification: the process of bringing together the child and family or previous caregiver for the purpose of establishing or re-establishing long-term care
- Follow-up: the term used to refer to a range of social and economic activities to facilitate the reintegration of the child within the family

Providing safe spaces

Often the first psychosocial support intervention in the midst of an emergency, a "Safe Space" (sometimes called "Child Friendly Spaces") program provides children with a structured and protective environment. The concept is simple and replicable: locate play space; identify, orient, and support community workers; mobilize groups of affected children; and, launch wide-scale play and recreation activities as soon as possible. Structured play and recreation helps normalize children's behavior at the very time they need it most. Safe Space programs also are readily scalable—using community resources, large numbers of children can be organized into these behavioral regulation programs in a short period of time. Although recreational and play activities (cooperative games, drawing, social drama, among others) are at the heart of the Safe Space concept, some programs have evolved into multifaceted intervention initiatives that eventually included immunization campaigns, nutrition programs, life skills activities, and parental support.

The humanitarian response to refugees in the aftermath of Rwanda's genocide provides an example of how Safe Space programs were taken to scale and laid the foundation for refugee education and a wider range of community support programs. It is also a case study of how the absence of Safe Space programs may undermine efforts to monitor child protection concerns.

In the spring of 1994, 250,000 Hutus fled to Tanzania in a single day to escape the repercussions of their leaders (and in many cases their own) involvement in the genocide in Rwanda. The humanitarian community responded to them as refugees in need of international assistance and protection. In a matter of weeks, 30,000 to 40,000 children were organized into Safe Space programs, with each group of children engaging in about 3 hours of structured activities per day. A "school-in-a-box" literary and numeracy program was added to this initial effort, providing children with a short-term learning opportunity as well as more structure to their day. These two psychosocial first-phase emergency responses paved the way for a more formal refugee education program and other community-based psychosocial support efforts. Indeed, a Safe Spaces program is an important step toward establishing curriculum-based learning in refugee or IDP situations where schools do not already exist.

Safe Space programs can provide needed psychosocial support as well as structures to monitor day-to-day protection concerns. The importance of Safe Spaces programs has been noted in postconflict redevelopment situations as well. In a report put forth by the Displaced Children's and Orphans Fund [58], for example, a lack of safe spaces was identified as an obstacle to an optimum path to psychosocial wellness among children in Afghanistan. The report further noted that the presence of minefields, rubble, and pollution played a factor in the absence of such facilities.

Relief agencies have developed basic guidelines for Safe Space programs in schools or other community locations [59]:

- The Safe Space program must be accessible to all, including children who have special needs.

- The safe space should be safe, and the facility (a tent will do) should be structurally and sound and able to protect children from the elements.
- The children must feel safe and secure from physical and/or sexual harassment, solicitation of drugs, weapons, and other dangerous materials.
- The safe space must be located in appropriate proximity to clean water and sanitation facilities.
- The safe space must be large enough to accommodate sports and recreation programs.

Mobilizing local beliefs and practices

Professional mental health services are nonexistent in majority of countries in which conflicts currently are taking place. In such settings, children's psychosocial well-being is linked to community self-help networks and local beliefs and practices [14,26,50]. Mobilizing these supports helps promote psychosocial healing and is key in reintegrating separated children, child soldiers, and other at-risk groups of girls and boys into families and communities.

One of the few longitudinal studies on war-affected children, for example, found that positive adult outcomes of former child soldiers were enhanced by community acceptance and traditional beliefs and practices [15]. In Mozambique, cleansing ceremonies date from precolonial times and are believed to be especially important when events such as war and population displacement upset the normal course of life. It is thought that the spirits of the victims of war will bring bad luck or death to the perpetrator and also to members of his extended family or community. Ancestor rebuke might come from simply missing a social duty or obligation toward others or might be triggered by contentious relationships among the living. Within this belief system, atrocities committed during the course of a brutal war become imbued with layers of spiritual meaning, necessitating such traditional ceremonies. These traditional practices afford individuals a chance to be cleansed of their acts during war and provide protection for the community from ancestral rebuke that might be brought on by the child's actions. Former child soldiers, family members, and neighbors cited cleansings ceremonies as vital for individual recovery and for rebuilding community trust and cohesion as well.

Future directions

War and political violence have direct effects on child development. Placing these many, varied effects within an ecologic framework is useful in two ways: it opens service providers' eyes to the many domains in which war and political violence may take their toll, and it illuminates the many elements of intervention necessary to protect children and enable them to cope more effectively. Three interventions—protection of separated children, provision of safe spaces, and mobilization of traditional healers and practices—have been identified as core psychosocial responses for children affected by armed conflict and forced migration.

As a field of practice, however, the provision of psychosocial care to children in crises is still in its infancy. Widely differing conceptual approaches—from addressing PTSD to reinforcing social support networks—have been adopted to justify interventions, but little evidence actually exists to support the efficacy of these approaches or to indicate how they might be employed to reinforce one another better. The international community still is largely unable to identify sufficient consensus regarding psychosocial goals, strategies, or outcomes. This lack of an evidence base for effective interventions undermines donor countries' confidence in psychosocial investments and leaves humanitarian workers wondering if their efforts made a difference.

Consistent and rigorous evaluations of program impact will be at the heart of efforts to professionalize this field of practice. In addition, children affected by conflict and displacement also would benefit from further insights into the following issues:

- How might the application of epidemiologic assessment approaches result in more timely and accurate identification of at-risk groups of children?
- What are the essential elements of effective programs to address PTSD, depression, and antisocial behavior?
- What are the most efficacious ways to address the psychologic and social needs of child soldiers and other groups of exploited girls and boys?
- Which social support mechanisms are instrumental in strengthening resilience and psychologic well-being?
- Which psychosocial approaches are scalable?

References

[1] Protecting refugees and the role of UNHCR. Geneva: United Nations High Commissioner for Refugees; 2007. Available at: http://www.unhcr.org/basics.html. Accessed January 4, 2008.
[2] Montgomery E, Foldspang A. Seeking asylum in Denmark: refugee children's mental health and exposure to violence. Eur J Public Health 2005;15(3):233–7.
[3] Machel G. The impact of war on children. Vancouver (Canada): UBC Press; 2001.
[4] Human rights watch stop child soldiers. Available at: http://www.humanrightswatch.org/campaigns/crp/where.htm. Accessed January 3, 2008.
[5] Boothby N, Ager A, Ager W. A guide to the evaluation of psychosocial programs in emergencies. New York: UNICEF; 2006.
[6] Forbes-Martin S. Policy perspective on mental health assistance to refugees. In: Marsella A, Borneman T, Ekblad E, editors. Amidst peril and pain: the mental health and well-being of the world's refugees. Washington, DC: American Psychological Association; 1994. p. 69–80.
[7] Baron N. Community-based psychosocial and mental health services for southern Sudanese refugees in long exile in Uganda. In: De Jong J, editor. Trauma, war and violence. New York: Kluwer; 2002. p. 157–203.

[8] Kostelny K, Wessells M. Internally displaced East Timorese: challenges and lessons of large-scale emergency assistance. In: Miller K, Rasco L, editors. The mental health of refugees: ecological approaches to healing and adaptation. Hillsdale (NJ): Erlbaum; 2004. p. 128–225.

[9] Honwana A. "Okusiakala Ondalo Yokalye": let us light a new fire. Local knowledge in the post-war healing and reintegration of war-affected children in Angola. Luanda (Angola): Christian Children's Fund/Angola; 1998.

[10] Honwana AM. Healing for peace: traditional healers and post-war reconstruction in southern Mozambique. Peace and Conflict: Journal of Peace Psychology 1997;3: 293–306.

[11] Honwana A. Non-Western concepts of mental health. In: Loughry M, Ager A, editors. The refugee experience, vol. 1Oxford (UK): Oxford University Refugee Studies Program; 1999. p. 103–19.

[12] Marsella A, Friedman M, Gerrity E, et al, editors. Ethno cultural aspects of posttraumatic stress disorder. Washington, DC: American Psychological Association; 1996.

[13] Nader K, Dubrow N, Stamm B, editors. Honoring differences: cultural issues in the treatment of trauma and loss. New York: Taylor and Francis; 1999.

[14] Wessells M. Child soldiers: from violence to protection. Cambridge (MA): Harvard University Press; 2006. p. 126–53.

[15] Boothby N, Crawford J, Halprin J. Mozambique child soldier life outcome study: lessons learned in rehabilitation and reintegration efforts. Global Public Health 2006;1:87–107.

[16] Arroyo W, Eth S. Post traumatic stress disorder and other stress responses. In: Apfel R, Simon B, editors. Minefields in their hearts. New Haven (CT): Yale University Press; 1996. p. 52–74.

[17] Fox S, Tang S. The Sierra Leonean refugee experience: traumatic events and psychiatric sequelae. J Nerv Ment Dis 2000;188:490–5.

[18] Hubbard J, Realmuto G, Northwood A, et al. Comorbidity of psychiatric diagnosis with posttraumatic stress disorder in survivors of childhood trauma. J Am Acad Child Adolesc Psychiatry 1995;34(9):1657–73.

[19] Miller K, Weine S, Ramic A, et al. The relative contribution of war experiences and exile-related stressors to levels of psychological distress among Bosnian refugees. J Trauma Stress 2002;15:377–87.

[20] Mollica R, McInnes K, Pham T, et al. The dose-effect relationships between torture and psychiatric symptoms in Vietnamese ex-political detainees and a comparison group. J Nerv Ment Dis 1998;186:543–53.

[21] Mollica R, Donelan K, Svang T, et al. The effect of trauma and confinement on functional health and mental health status of Cambodians living in Thailand-Cambodia border camps. JAMA 1993;27:581–6.

[22] De Jong J. Public mental health, traumatic stress and human rights violation in low income countries. In: De Jong J, editor. Trauma, war and violence: public mental health in socio-cultural context. New York: Kluwer Academic/Plenum Publishers; 2002. p. 1–92.

[23] Smith P, Perrin S, Yule W, et al. War exposure among children from Bosnia-Herzegovina: psychological adjustment in a community sample. J Trauma Stress 2002;15:147–56.

[24] Thabet A, Vostanis P. Post-traumatic stress disorder reactions in children of war: a longitudinal study. Child Abuse Negl 2000;24:291–8.

[25] Garbarino J, Kostelny K. The effects of political violence on Palestinian children's behavior problems: a risk accumulation model. Child Dev 1996;67:33–45.

[26] Boothby N, Strang A, Wessells M, editors. A world turned upside down: social ecological approaches to children in war zones. Bloomfield (CT): Kumarian Press; 2006.

[27] De Jong J. Public mental health, traumatic stress and human rights violation in low income countries. In: De Jong J, editor. Trauma, war and violence: Public mental health in socio-cultural context. New York (NY): Kluwer Academic/Plenum Publishers; 2002. p. 1–92.

[28] Dyregov A, Yule W. Screening measures—the development of the UNICEF screening battery. Presented at the Symposium on War-Affected Children in former Yugoslavia at the

Eleventh Annual Meeting of the International Society for Traumatic Stress Studies. Boston; November, 1995.

[29] Gibson K. Children in political violence. Soc Sci Med 1989;7:659–67.

[30] Dawes A. The effects of political violence on children: a consideration of South African and related studies. Int J Psychol 1990;25:13–31.

[31] Punamaki R, Suleiman R. Predictors and effectiveness of coping with political violence among Palestinian children. Br J Soc Psychol 1990;29:67–77.

[32] Kostelny K. A culture-based, integrative approach. In: Boothby N, Strang A, Wessells M, editors. A world turned upside down: sociological approaches to children in war zones. Bloomfield (CT): Kumarian Press, Inc.; 2006. p. 19–38.

[33] Ressler E, Boothby N, Steinbock D. Unaccompanied children in emergencies: care and protection in wars, natural disasters and mass population movements. New York: Oxford University Press; 1988. p. 153–73.

[34] Frazer M. Children in conflict. New York: Basic Books; 1973.

[35] Garbarino J, Kostelny K, Dubrow N. No place to be a child: growing up in a war zone. Lexington (MA): Lexington Books; 1991.

[36] Sameroff A, Seifer R, Barocas R, et al. Intelligence quotient scores of 4-year-old children: social environmental risk factors. Pediatrics 1987;79:343–50.

[37] Macksoud MS, Aber JL. The war experiences and psychosocial development of children in Lebanon. Child Dev 1996;67:70–88.

[38] Bronfenbrenner U. The ecology of human development. Experiments by nature and design. Cambridge (MA): Harvard University Press; 1979.

[39] Bronfenbrenner U. Ecology of the family as a context for human development: research perspectives. Dev Psychol 1986;22:732–42.

[40] Bracken P. Hidden agendas: deconstructing post-traumatic stress disorder. In: Brachen P, Petty C, editors. Rethinking the trauma of war. London: Free Association Books; 1998. p. 38–59.

[41] Wessells M. Culture, power, and community: intercultural approaches to psychosocial assistance and healing. In: Nader K, Dubrow N, Stamm B, editors. Honoring differences: cultural issues in the treatment of trauma and loss. New York: Taylor and Francis; 1999. p. 276–82.

[42] Rugh A. Home-based girls' schools in Balochistan refugee villages: a strategy study: save the children. Save the Children USA Pakistan/Afghanistan Field Office; 2000.

[43] Boothby N, Ager A, Wessells M, et al. How do we know what works in protection: building the evidence base. Care and protection of children in crisis-affected countries project. Washington, DC: Presentation to the Washington Network on Children and Armed Conflict; 2007.

[44] Bremer M, Ager A, Boothby N. Situation analysis of child protection in Darfur. United Nations Children's Fund; 2006; in press.

[45] Rutter M. Resilience in the face of adversity: protective factors and resistance to psychological disorder. Br J Psychiatry 1985;147:598–611.

[46] Lewis M, Lockheed M. Getting all girls into schools. Finance and development. vol. 44 (No 2). Washington, DC: International Monetary Fund; 2007.

[47] Wessells M, Monteiro C. Psychosocial assistance to internally displaced people in Angola: a child focused, community-based approach. In: Miller K, Rasco LM, editors. From clinic to community: ecological approaches to refugee mental health. Upper Saddle River (NJ): Erlbaum; 2004. p. 67–94.

[48] Ahearn F. Psychosocial wellness: methodological approaches to the study of refugees. In: Ahearn F, editor. Psychosocial wellness of refugees. New York: Berghahn; 2000. p. 3–23.

[49] Boothby N. Mobilizing communities to meet the psychosocial needs of children in war and refugee situations. In: Apfel R, Simon B, editors. Minefields in their hearts. New Haven (CT): Yale University Press; 1996. p. 52–74.

[50] Gibbs S. Postwar social reconstruction in Mozambique: reframing children's experiences of trauma and healing. In: Kumar K, editor. Rebuilding war-torn societies: critical areas for international assistance. Boulder (CO): Lynne Rienner; 1997. p. 227–38.

[51] Wessells M, Monteiro C. Psychosocial interventions and post-war reconstruction in Angola: interweaving western and traditional approaches. In: Christie D, Wagner RV, Winter D, editors. Peace, conflict, and violence: peace psychology for the 21st century. Upper Saddle River (NJ): Prentice-Hall; 2001. p. 262–75.

[52] Brown M. Family tracing and reunification case study: Rwanda. In: Brown M, Charnley H, Petty C, editors. Children separated by war: family tracing and reunification. Save the Children Conference report. London: Save the Children UK; 1995.

[53] Tolfree D. Community based care for separated children. Stockholm (Sweden): Save the Children Sweden; 2003.

[54] Inter-Agency Guiding Principles on Unaccompanied and Separated Children (IGAP). Geneva (Switzerland): International Committee of the Red Cross, United Nations High Commissioner for Refugees, United Nations Children's Fund, International Rescue Committee, Save the Children UK, World Vision International; 2003.

[55] Hepburn A, Williamson J, Wolfram T. Separated children: care and protection of children in emergencies—a field guide. Save the children; US children in crisis field guide series. New York: Save the Children Federation; 2004.

[56] Dona G. The Rwandan experience of fostering separated children. Stockholm (Sweden): Save the Children Sweden; 2001.

[57] Sprenkels R. Lives apart: family separation and alternative care arrangements during El Salvador's civil war. Stockholm (Sweden): Save the Children Sweden; 2002.

[58] USAID-funded Child Protection and Psychosocial Support for Afghan Children and Youth Project. Displaced Children's and Orphans Fund. Third quarterly project report. Oct–Dec 2003.

[59] Child protection. United Nations Children's Fund, 2004. Available at: http://www.unicef.org/teachers/protection/instability.htm. Accessed January 3, 2008.

ELSEVIER
SAUNDERS

Child Adolesc Psychiatric Clin N Am
17 (2008) 515–532

CHILD AND
ADOLESCENT
PSYCHIATRIC CLINICS
OF NORTH AMERICA

Family Roles in Refugee Youth Resettlement from a Prevention Perspective

Stevan Weine, MD

*Department of Psychiatry, College of Medicine, University of Illinois
at Chicago, 1601 W. Taylor Street, Room 589, Chicago, IL 60612, USA*

Where is the refugee family?

Service providers from many different fields who are working with resettled refugees are committed to making their hometowns great cities of refuge. They extend helping hands to the newcomers, no matter where they come from, what language they speak, their race, or religion. They pick new arrivals up at airports, find apartments for them, familiarize newly settled refugees with their new city, get them jobs, teach them English, give them health and mental health care, and teach their children.

In particular, the providers reach out to refugee children. Sometimes these children are old for their years, but they still are open to the new circumstances and are looking for helping hands. Many times, one or both of the youths' parents are not there, or the parents are too occupied with work or their own adjustments to a new world and a new way of life. A practice pattern has been established in refugee services that responds to refugee children loosened from their families and targets children rather than their less-reachable parents or the family as a whole. This pattern is called "youth services," "psychosocial services," or "mental health interventions."

Although this youth-focused practice pattern has benefited some refugee youth and adults, it also has limitations. One particular concern is that it may overlook the role of the family in the lives of resettling refugee youth—"overlook" in the sense that it intervenes primarily with youth and does not seek to make changes in the family system or the families' interactions with communities, organizations, or other families. Refugee families,

---

E-mail address: smweine@uic.edu

despite the losses, separations, or traumas they have suffered, still are the primary social context for resettled refugee youth. As such, refugee service providers should not overlook families.

Some helping professionals in the refugee services field, such as family therapists, have kept a focus on the family. The perspective and activities of family therapists can be found in the family therapy literature on refugee families, including families from Central American, the Balkans, and Asia. This literature is largely the product of therapeutic activities and applied family theory rather than systematic research. Family therapy has tended to focus on family conflicts that result from the interaction of unprocessed traumatic experiences and on intergenerational stresses stemming from adjustment in the resettlement context [1]. These issues include "relational and emotional conflicts" in which previously functional patterns of behavior within families are found not to work well within the resettlement setting. Consider, for example, how traditional cultural values and patriarchal gender roles are challenged in the resettlement context by a more liberal cultural environment that has different expectations and in which there is a financial need for women to work outside the home [2].

Although the family therapy perspective on refugees makes clinically accurate and helpful observations, at times it may be somewhat biased toward identifying family conflicts and less attuned to family strengths. This potential bias leads one to ask whether the family conflicts actually are as prevalent, intense, or significant as this literature indicates. There also is some risk for any service provider to view family conflicts as inherent properties of a family rather than as sequelae of the social and economic conditions thrust upon these families. Even though family therapists know to look for family cultural strengths (eg, extended families, family obligations, religious faith), when the traumas, losses, and strains on refugee families are so great, there is a risk that service providers will not sufficiently comprehend or acknowledge the resources and strengths that lie within families [3].

The author and his colleagues have been conducting a program of research focused on the prevention of mental disorders and behavioral problems in refugee families (The meaning of prevention is defined later in this article). At this juncture, it should be noted that, in comparison with family therapy, family-focused prevention places less emphasis on identifying what is broken in families that may need to be fixed therapeutically. Instead, the emphasis is more on identifying family strengths and resources that can be enhanced through preventive interventions so as to address better the strains on the family and the risks posed to youths' functioning [2]. As a research-based approach, family-focused prevention endeavors to base prevention strategies on a systematic characterization of both the strains and the strengths of refugee families through research, including the use of ethnographic methods.

Strains on refugee families

Our family has not been together since we fled our village. My brother was killed, and two of our children went with his wife into the jungle and ended up in a different camp. When the officials came to interview us at the refugee camp for coming to the United States, they asked for our papers and had us draw a family tree. They thought we might be lying, but we cannot help it if we don't think the same as they about who is in our family. They gave us cultural orientation, which was real nice, but one thing that we did not like was when they said that we could not discipline our children, and that if we did we would be put in jail or deported. What will happen to our children if they do not know right and wrong? That was only the beginning of the changes to our family. Here, the children are going places, making friends, and having a better life. All we do is work, worry about bills, worry about sending money back home, and if we are ever going to see the rest of our family. Our life here is not how they said it was going to be, and there is nothing my wife and I can do to make it better.

Refugee families may enter resettlement having suffered major family traumas, losses, or separations caused by political violence and forced displacement or even by the manner in which they were processed through the refugee resettlement system. This system may have a way of defining the family and its members that is different from how these families think of themselves as a family. One example is that families from cultures that practice polygamy must divide into nuclear families, each of which may be resettled in different cities or countries. Similarly, families from cultures that are not accustomed to distinguishing between sons/daughters and nephews/nieces also may be separated, because the system for resettling refugees is based on the Western construct of the nuclear family.

Refugee families, like other immigrants, come with expectations of a better life in America. Their expectations of America have been nurtured by word of mouth from friends and family, Hollywood movies, and the overseas cultural orientation sessions funded by the US Department of State's Bureau of Population, Refugees, and Migration and implemented by one of several nongovernmental organizations. When they first arrive in resettlement locations in the United States, most refugee families find themselves living in poverty in urban areas, working low-wage jobs that require that both parents be income earners, and having less time than they are accustomed to spend with their family [4]. In addition to the traumas and losses that the families experienced in their home countries or in flight, resettlement conditions subject them to further strain.

The author and colleagues' prior research with refugees from Bosnia-Herzegovina has documented multiple areas of family life in which members of refugee families reported adverse consequences resulting from war, forced displacement, exile, and urbanization [5]. They reported multiple changes in family roles and obligations, including living through their children, having less family time, and challenges to a patriarchal family system. Families that survived political violence often lived with traumatic memories linked to those experiences, and these memories could complicate family communication. Families reported changes in their relationship with other family members, such as now being part of transnational families, with other family members living either in their home country or in other countries of exile. Family members were concerned about changes in their connections with the ethnic community and nation state, citing concerns about children becoming Americanized and losing touch with traditional ways of life.

Although refugee children are not equivalent to immigrant children, given the substantial overlap, it is pertinent to consider that quantitative research on immigrant children has identified several statistically significant factors that make adjustment more difficult: (1) less-educated parents; (2) low-wage work with no benefits; (3) no English-speaking adults in the home; (4) family poverty; (5) lack of supports to the family; and (6) discrimination and racism against family members [6].

Other sources of difficulty for refugee families that deserve further mention pertain to particular areas of cultural difference. Families that come from cultures that practice corporal punishment are told in cultural orientation sessions both overseas and in the United States that such behaviors will be considered child abuse and that they may be subject to jail or deportation [7]. These families are challenged to devise other approaches to child discipline, but as a consequence often feel powerless to control their children's behaviors. Another important area of cultural difference concerns adolescents [8]. For families from many cultures in which traditionally there is no prolonged transitional period between childhood and adulthood, the idea of a youth becoming a "teenager" often is a new cultural construct. When refugee youth start to behave like American teenagers, refugee parents often are unsure how to respond. In particular, they are unfamiliar with the kind of parental monitoring and supervision that parents need to provide to help their teenagers stay safe in urban America.

Family resources and strengths

> The reason that our people have survived so much hardship is because of our families. We believe very much in families, and we work to keep them strong. Everybody has a place in the family, and they know where they belong. They know that they can always count on others in the family to help them if they have a problem. Our families tie together male and female, and young and old, across the generations and even over the centuries. Our families have lots of faith and keep us close to God. If you visit any of our houses, you can see that we try to make it a place where all of us feel comfortable and like to be together. Just being together gives us all great pleasure.

Although the emphasis placed on the strains of refugee families is certainly supported by facts, the existence of strengths is just as real and

important a dimension in their lives. The author and colleagues' prior research with Bosnian refugee families in the United States has documented
multiple areas of family life in which family members report engaging in
helpful responses to the aforementioned strains [5]. Families have found
ways to manage the changes in family roles and obligations. These methods
include letting children provide hope; fostering flexibility, tolerance, and
trust in the family; and promoting family togetherness. Families manage difficulties in communication by sharing good memories, talking with children,
and expressing their emotions. Refugee families respond to changes in relationships with other family members through several strategies—such as
sending money home, planning an eventual return, and maintaining a transnational family—that help maintain a sense of connectedness with the larger
family and its members. To cope with changes in their connection with the
ethnic community and nation state, family members adopt several strategies,
including teaching children the history and language of their country of
origin and strengthening ethnocultural identity.

The quantitative impact of family strengths on refugee youth is not well
studied. A number of small and mostly cross-sectional quantitative studies
have identified possible protective resources, such as family support [9,10],
parental well-being and lower caregiver distress [11], family connection to
the large community/social support, family connections to the culture of
origin [12], and affirmation through shared experience [13]. Also of interest,
research on immigrant youth has identified the following family-related
characteristics that impact youth adaptation: (1) healthy, intact families;
(2) strong work ethic and aspirations; and (3) community cohesion [14].

The domain of culture, which, as previously stated poses difficulties for
refugees, is also associated with strengths. Commonly cited strengths documented in the author and colleagues' research include a sense of obligation
to family, a work ethic, and support from the same ethnic community [15].
Research with refugees has indicated that a stronger cultural identity may
play a protective role regarding mental health outcomes [16]. Family
research in other populations has demonstrated that family stories, family
rituals, and family routines are associated with changes in family processes
and improved health behaviors and health outcomes [17]. Although this
type of research has not yet been conducted with refugee families, findings
from several ethnographic studies conducted by the author and colleagues
have shown how refugee families are able to draw on some of these existing
family cultural scripts whereas others must be converted in order to be useful in the new surroundings.

Family-focused interventions with refugees

From necessity, some providers of psychosocial services to refugees have
developed patterns for how they work with refugee families. Family therapists, for example, have conducted family assessments, provided brief or

long-term family therapy to address issues of family conflict, or provided family therapy consultation regarding mental health or health problems of individual family members. Family therapists' work with refugee families usually is provided through refugee resettlement agencies, refugee mental health programs, schools, or faith-based organizations.

Alternatively, multiple-family groups have been used in working with refugee families to provide family support and education and to facilitate access to mental health services and other community-based services. The author and colleagues' research program designed, implemented, and evaluated several multiple-family group interventions with Bosnian and Kosovar refugees in Chicago. The first such intervention, with Bosnian refugees, was known as "CAFES" (for Coffee and Family Education and Support). CAFES was a community-based, time-limited, multiple-family education and support group for survivors who had posttraumatic stress disorder (PTSD) and their families. Longitudinal assessments showed that CAFES was effective as an access intervention for mental health services [18]. The investigators then adapted CAFES for a focus on families of early and middle adolescents, called "Youth CAFES," designed to improve parenting and the parent-youth relationship, and conducted a feasibility pilot with qualitative assessments [19]. Next, they adapted CAFES for newly re-settled adult refugees from Kosovo, designing a "TAFES" (for Tea and Families Education and Support) group. The uncontrolled postintervention assessments demonstrated increases in social support and use of psychiatric services and improvements over time in scale scores assessing trauma mental health knowledge, trauma mental health attitudes, and family hardiness [20]. Researchers working with Hispanic migrants also have developed multiple-family group interventions to diminish the acculturation gap between parents and children. For example, Szapocznik and colleagues [21] developed and evaluated the Bicultural Effectiveness Training for Hispanic youth and families.

Other types of family interventions being used with refugees come from the family-strengthening movement, which has spawned the development of family education initiatives [22]. In the refugee field, these interventions focus primarily on parenting and marriage education [22,23]. At present family-strengthening interventions with refugees are largely donor-driven initiatives and practice-based programs that apply models that have been used in the general population to refugee populations on a trial-and-error basis. At this point, these initiatives do not evaluate their family-focused interventions systematically.

Refugee families have areas of cultural difference from the host community, organizations, and providers, so cultural issues complicate these efforts at family intervention with refugees. For example, refugees and interveners may have different understandings regarding the definition of the family. Thus, providers for refugee families face the difficult challenge of adapting interventions from one cultural context to another. Unfortunately, there has been little systematic study to identify which constructs are applicable across sociocultural contexts and which are group specific. The issue of translating intervention strategies is a major challenge for both prevention and treatment in refugee services. Given the increasing number of immigrants and refugees in the United States population, intervention adaptation and translation has become a growing concern in mental health services research [24].

Need for family-centered preventive interventions

> Overall far more is known about PTSD than about how young people manage to survive, adjust, and prosper. Far more is known about the clinical treatment of PTSD in refugee youth than how to design, implement, and evaluate preventive interventions that include a focus on their families and communities.

In the 1980s, to improve prevention efforts among state mental health programs for refugees, the National Institute of Mental Health and the Office of Refugee Resettlement funded a project to integrate the research on refugee mental health with the primary prevention of psychopathology [25]. It produced reports calling for the development of preventive interventions to address mental health problems in refugees, especially children [26]. None were developed, because at the time institutional priorities favored either individually oriented clinical services or large-scale preventive intervention studies (S. Williams, personal communication, 2005). With the arrival of increasing numbers of new refugees and their known psychosocial needs, there is now greater interest in developing preventive interventions for refugees. In addition, the limitations of youth-targeted clinical approaches are becoming more apparent to policymakers, scientists, and front-line workers.

Although there has been little prevention work in the field of trauma mental health, the concept of prevention has been discussed recently in relation to disaster preparedness and early intervention [27]. The major report of the World Health Organization (WHO) on prevention of mental disorders uses the following framework [28]:

Primary prevention encompasses
1. Selective prevention, which targets individuals or subgroups at elevated risk for a mental disorder because of risk factors (eg, exposure to trauma)
2. Indicated prevention, which targets persons at high risk who have minimal but detectable signs or symptoms (eg, traumatic stress symptoms)
   Secondary prevention seeks to lower the rate of established disorders (eg, PTSD) through early detection and treatment
   Tertiary prevention seeks to reduce disability, enhance rehabilitation, and prevent relapse and recurrence.

The WHO recommended that preventive interventions in trauma mental health might focus on any of these different points, separately or together.

The WHO and the Institute of Medicine also have spoken of mental disorder prevention, which aims at "reducing incidence, prevalence, and recurrence of mental disorders, the time spent with symptoms, or the risk condition for a mental illness, preventing or delaying recurrences and also decreasing the impact of illness in the affected person, their families and the society" [28,29]. These frameworks can be used as starting points to inform the development of preventive interventions for refugee families.

Through a prevention approach, services may be able to enhance protective resources so as to stop, lessen, or delay possible mental health and behavioral sequelae in youth, such as PTSD, depression, substance abuse, and school problems [30]. Given the high costs of treatment and of untreated conditions, effective preventive interventions probably would be cost saving. There are important protective resources within refugee families that may be harnessed toward prevention if they can be identified [31,32].

Multiple indicators suggest the need to broaden the concept of prevention with refugee youth beyond PTSD and even diagnosable mental disorders. Refugee providers routinely document a range of diagnosable disorders, such as depression, anxiety, substance abuse, and behavioral problems including HIV/AIDS risk behaviors, early pregnancy, and school problems [15,17,33]. Researchers recognize that the refugee field has been focused too exclusively on the etiologic significance of war trauma and now seeks to place more emphasis on stresses associated with forced migration and on other contextual variables, such as discrimination or gender and power differentials. Services researchers recognize that little is known about how trauma services operate in different cultural and organizational contexts [34]. In addition, little research has examined trauma systematically from a family perspective (eg, family as a context) both for risk (eg, parental mental illness) and protection (eg, parental support). All these factors have important implications for developing targeted preventive interventions for refugee families.

Another important impetus for developing preventive interventions is that, although many youth are suffering, most do not seek mental health services. Among refugees, the stigma related to mental illness and seeking mental health services often is very high [35,36]. Experience with refugees from Africa and Asia suggests that greater degrees of cultural difference are associated with even greater stigma and higher barriers to the use of mental health services [33,37]. Preventive interventions are needed because they offer paths for reaching persons who are difficult to reach through clinical interventions [38].

A family resilience perspective on refugees

Building preventive interventions for refugee youth calls for further developing a family resilience perspective on refugee youth and their families. A family resilience perspective claims that the family is a key context for refugee youth. Refugee youth live in families in which multiple traumas and losses may interact with social and economic difficulties, cultural transitions, and possible parental mental illness. Still, their families also contain resources and strengths that may be protective against negative outcomes for youth. To deploy these resources and strengths effectively in their new circumstances, families may need additional knowledge, skills, relationships, or practice.

Because families do not function in isolation, a family resilience conceptualization also encompasses ecologic protective resources, such as those involving the school and community. The theoretic underpinning of this view of family resilience is family eco-developmental theory, which envisions youth in the context of a family system that interacts with larger social systems [39,40].

Prevention researchers working with nonrefugee populations have studied resilience-based family and school intervention programs and have found that effective preventive interventions build on existing protective resources associated with families and communities [28,41]. For example, Beardslee [42,43] developed and evaluated a family-oriented preventive intervention for youth of parents who had affective illness and demonstrated improvements in understanding, coping strategies, and functioning in families. Strategies learned from the implementation of effective resilience programs may be applied to preventive interventions with refugees. For example, family-focused interventions may be more effective than strictly child- or parent-focused strategies, but this requires that these interventions are tailored to the cultural traditions of the families [29,44].

In a related area of research, research in developmental psychopathology has focused on the resilience of children facing poverty, alcoholism, physical illness, and mental illness [45,46]. Werner's empirically derived conceptual model specifies five clusters of protective factors: (1) "temperamental characteristics"; (2) "skills and values that lead to efficient use of whatever abilities they had"; (3) "parental caregiving that fostered child self-esteem"; (4) "supportive adults who fostered trust and were gatekeeper to the future"; and (5) "opening of opportunities at major life transitions" [47,48]. Other researchers have identified within-family protective factors such as supportive parent–child relationships, positive discipline methods, monitoring and supervision, and advocacy for children [49,50]. The challenge in applying these research findings to developing preventive interventions that are focused on family resilience is to reconceptualize protective factors not as static properties but as active family processes that directly or indirectly facilitate positive youth outcomes and that can be modified through interventions.

Focus on the family role in education: problems and approaches to prevention

It is hard for me to talk with my parents about the problems that I am having at school. They don't understand the system here, and it is

completely different from the system in our country. The only time my
mother has been to school was to pick up the report cards. My father
doesn't go. They are both too busy with work, and because of the language
problem they can't communicate. Ever since the school put me in the
wrong grade, I've had so many problems. The programmer just put me
there, and there was nothing I could say. They give me homework which
I don't understand. My parents think that if it was a better school, it
would finish everything there and not need to send all this work home.
They don't like my friends and the new way I cut my hair. I know they
care, but when they yell it makes things worse. I guess that's why some
of my friends stopped going to school.

To deepen this discussion of family roles in refugee youth resettlement
from a prevention perspective, one area of concern is considered in greater
detail: the role of parents in youth's education. Parental involvement may be
defined as the active participation of parents, both in school and at home, to
support their children's educational achievement [51]. This topic has been
chosen because, although many refugee youth do exceedingly well at school,
many, unfortunately, do not.

There is little published research on the refuge parents' involvement in
youths' education. A study of Hmong refugee families showed that parents
viewed the teachers as the experts and did not expect to be involved [52]. A
study of Khmer parents found low parental involvement in youths' education, and parents explained that they did not see it as in their role to push
their children to achieve [53]. Studies of Russian refugee families report conflicts between parents and children over youth not studying enough [54].
These findings are of concern, because existing research from nonrefugee
populations suggests that parental involvement in education is associated
with improved outcomes for youth (eg, educational achievement, behavioral
improvement, and longer-term functioning), for parents (eg, improved attitudes, advocacy, and community ties), and for schools (eg, improved teacher
morale and school performance) [55,56]. Could inadequate parental involvement of refugee parents be part of the explanation for school problems
among refugee youth?

All refugee parents say they want their children to have a better life in
their new country, but, understandably, they may have difficulties converting these hopes into educational involvement that is effective in the new
context. After all, refugee parents differ in their prior experiences with
education. For example, those who come from rural settings often have
lower levels of formal education. Refugee families also differ in how
much emphasis they currently place on education as a means of improving
their children's lives [57]. It is common to hear refugee parents say that
education is important because it leads to better jobs. If you ask them
whether by "education" they mean high school or college, they almost
always reply, "College." Too often, however, parents have very little familiarity with primary and secondary schools in the United States, let alone

colleges. Given the intense financial pressures upon these families, it is not surprising that many refugee youth are encouraged by their parents to work full or part time while attending high school. However, this can further diminish youth and parental emphasis on education.

Parents in refugee families face many obstacles to involvement in their children's education: illiteracy, not speaking English, heavy work schedules, being unaccustomed to active school involvement, a sense of embarrassment about their children's performance or conduct, and unfamiliarity with how to support their child's education. In many refugee parents' prior societies, parental involvement in their children's education was viewed as interfering and disrespectful. Some schools that work with refugees and immigrants have developed helpful strategies for addressing these impediments: making information available to parents in their home language, inviting parents to participate in special activities, and encouraging parent-to-teacher liaison [58]. Nonetheless, the impediments that refugee parents face regarding involvement usually are greater than the schools' or resettlement organizations' strategies of response. For example, both regular and bilingual teachers may not receive adequate training, support, or resources to work with refugee students and families.

From a family resilience perspective, parental involvement in education may be considered a protective factor for refugee youth that could have a potentially high impact on the youth and the family in multiple realms of individual and family functioning. In addition to facilitating school achievement for youth, parental involvement in education may be associated with other youth-level outcomes, such as improved youth mental health outcomes, youth peer relations, and youth employment and earning capacity. Parental involvement in education also may facilitate family-level changes including family advocacy for youth, family communication, family integration in communities, and family contact with other families. Last, parental involvement can promote school-level changes, such as teachers and administrators gaining a greater familiarity with refugee families, better communication with their students' parents, and better collaborative partnership with parents in planning refugee children's education [56].

Of course parental involvement in education is not the only protective factor that has been identified for refugee youth. In comparison with others, such as mentoring or family stories and rituals, however, it may be the one that has the broadest reach. This possibility suggests that parental involvement in education would serve well as a primary aim of preventive interventions with refugee youth.

At present, parental involvement in education receives some attention from resettlement organizations and from schools. For example, in initial cultural orientation sessions and ongoing parenting classes, refugee parents are informed about schools and encouraged to become involved in their children's education. In schools with substantial numbers of refugees and bilingual programs, the bilingual coordinator or bilingual teachers may make special efforts to reach out to refugee parents. Schools also may have a bilingual parent council or cultural events that attempt to engage with refugee families. Despite these valuable efforts, providers involved with refugee youth have expressed concern that parental involvement in education still is not being addressed sufficiently by schools, voluntary agencies, or communities.

A particular concern is that achieving parental involvement in education may require a level of change within the families that is beyond the scope of the aforementioned agency- or school-based efforts. That is, making significant changes in the attitudes, roles, and behaviors of parents with respect to involvement in their children's education may require more than new information alone. For example, programs may consider aiming to modify the educational goals and aspirations of refugee youth and parents. Another concern is that the types of activities that parents need to undertake for involvement in youths' education may require fairly intensive skills training. For example, some existing parental involvement programs focus on increasing the parents' ability to ask appropriate questions of the teacher, increasing the parent's ability to help their youth doing homework, and increasing parent-to-parent interaction [59,60]. Helping some refugee parents achieve these tasks can be quite challenging.

Although no known preventive interventions to improve parental involvement in education have been tested in refugees, many different interventions have been evaluated in nonrefugee populations. Furthermore, although there are concerns about the quality of the research methodology (eg, whether it adequately considers adolescent developmental processes), and some of the results are mixed, there are promising findings regarding certain approaches, including school outreach to families; respecting and understanding cultural differences among families; and building trust through family, school, and community collaborative relationships [56].

Applying family eco-developmental theory also suggests that interventions that aim to promote parental involvement should target the school and community as well as the parents. Consistent with that view, some existing parental involvement programs focus on (1) improving teachers' abilities to work with immigrant parents; (2) improving the school's accessibility to immigrant parents by offering other services; and (3) improving the school's engagement with the community by participating in or hosting community activities [58].

Of course, several important questions concerning a preventive intervention to increase parental involvement in education have yet to be answered:

Who should conduct the intervention and where?
What are the specific aims and methods of the intervention?
How would the intervention target different age groups (eg, preadolescents versus adolescents)?
How would the intervention need to vary across different refugee groups?

Further research on refugee families, schools, and communities, including preventive intervention trials, are needed to answer these questions. Nonetheless, it is hard to escape the conclusion that there is a need to develop prevention interventions that promote parental involvement in education for refugee youth. This effort should be undertaken by those who share the responsibility for promoting parent involvement with refugees, including communities, schools and school districts, resettlement agencies, and the state.

Collaboration with families and communities

> Parental involvement is a Western middle class idea. We didn't have nothing like that in our country. Involvement meant that you didn't show respect for the authority of the teachers. We would never want to show that.

When asking parents or families to change their behaviors, it helps to know what these behaviors mean to them and what beliefs or experiences underlie these behaviors. Parental involvement in education, for example, is a construct that will vary according to sociocultural context and that can be addressed best through an inquiry based on partnership between researchers and families and communities. For example, if an intervention aims to modify youth and parental goals and aspirations for education (eg, setting higher goals), then partnership in designing that intervention would help assure that the intervention respected and drew upon important family resources and strengths. This is one reason for using a community-based participatory research (CBPR) approach, defined later, to the development of preventive interventions for refugee families. Another indication for CBPR is that refugee families and communities may have justifiable problems trusting service providers, researchers, and their respective organizations, given prior experiences with traumas and betrayals [34]. Interventions will not succeed unless first adequate trust is established.

In the author and colleagues' approach to family preventive interventions, informed by CBPR, adult and youth family and community members and other key community stakeholders are partners in each phase of the work from conception to dissemination of results. Key CBPR principles [61,62] include:

1. Building on cultural and community strengths (eg, family values)
2. Colearning among all community and research partners
3. Shared decision making
4. Commitment to applying findings with the goal of improving health by taking action, including social change
5. Mutual ownership of the research process and products

The author and colleagues believe that a CBPR approach is necessary to address the specific mental health challenges in refugee families and communities. Most important is giving families, youth, schools, and community leaders a real voice in the development and implementation of interventions. Also essential is fostering collaborations with community health, mental health, and scientific institutions. Thus, a CBPR approach should (1) make the voices of refugee youth and parents heard and relevant to services and science; (2) increase the confidence and competence of parents, community-based providers, educators, and leaders; and (3) build a learning system that keeps knowledge flowing and communication open between these families, communities, schools, organizations, and researchers.

Each refugee community is likely to have its own needs, meanings, strengths, and preferences. These qualities would be expected to inform the prioritization of concerns and their opinions about what problems require what types of interventions. Thus, it is potentially complicated but nevertheless important to give refugee communities the opportunity to introduce these issues into the design, implementation, and evaluation of interventions. Unfortunately, investigating this type of complexity does not lend itself easily to testing the effectiveness of an intervention through a randomized, controlled trial. However, newer models, such as the comprehensive dynamic trial methodology, may be appropriate [63].

Need for focus on engaging refugee families

> The group sounds good, but it's hard for us to get there. My husband works days, and I go to work at four, just after the children come home from school. If it's on the weekend, which is the only time we have to be at home as a family. We don't know all these other families and they don't know us. To get there, we would have to pay for the transportation. I don't know, maybe we'd give it a try. It might help if it were on a Sunday. Should we bring our small children?

Even the best preventive intervention does no good if the invited participants do not come to the meetings. On any given day, refugee families have many obstacles that would keep them from attending any type of psychosocial intervention. Some of these barriers are practical (eg, transportation and babysitting), and some are more existential (eg, a belief that what is happening in a family should stay in a family). The impediments to participating in a preventive intervention are especially strong, because parents and other family members do not necessarily see themselves as having a problem for which they need immediate help. Therefore preventive interventions with refugee families require specific strategies for engagement.

The author and colleagues' prior studies of engagement with Bosnian refugee families demonstrated that they were effective in engaging (73%) and retaining (83%) family members [64]. The findings indicated that families that engaged in a multiple-family support and education group had experienced significantly more transitions, more traumas, and more difficulties in adjustment than those who did not engage. Engagement also was related to family member's perceptions about strategies for responding to adversities.

Families that engaged had concerns about traumatic memories that persisted despite their avoidant behaviors; however, they were even more concerned about keeping the family together, supporting their children, and rebuilding their social life. This study underlined the importance of a focus on engagement in conducting preventive interventions with refugee families. It suggested that the strategies for engaging refugee families in multiple-family groups should correspond to the particular ways that the targeted families manage transitions, traumas, and adjustment difficulties.

Overall, the author and colleagues have found that a family prevention program requires spending at least as much effort in engaging families as it does in conducting the intervention itself. The first step in engagement is understanding the primary concerns of the parents and the youth. The author and colleagues have developed engagement scripts, based upon ethnographic research and community and family collaboration, which group facilitators or other recruiters can use to talk with families about the group. These scripts clarify for families that this group is focused on the areas of concern that they and most refugee families have. The script also specifically describe the obstacles to their participation and achievable steps for overcoming these obstacles. Once a family comes to the first group, sees other families that share the same difficulties, and hears that the group leaders want to help them draw on family strengths to address today's and tomorrow's challenges, they will commit to working together.

Acknowledgment

The author gratefully acknowledges the support of the National Institute of Mental Health (R01 MH076118-02).

References

[1] McGoldrick M, Giordano J, Garcia-Preto N. Ethnicity and family therapy. New York: The Guilford Press; 2005.
[2] McGoldrick M. Re-visioning family therapy. New York: The Guilford Press; 1998.
[3] Walsh F. Strengthening family resilience. New York: Guilford Press; 1998.
[4] Lustig S, Kia-Keating M, Grant-Knight W, et al. Review of child and adolescent refugee mental health. J Am Acad Child Adolesc Psychiatry 2004;43:24–39.
[5] Weine SM, Muzurovic N, Kulauzovic Y, et al. Family consequences of political violence in refugee families. Fam Process 2004;43:147–60.
[6] Fuligni AJ. Adolescents from immigrant families. In: McLoyd VC, Steinberg L, editors. Studying minority adolescents: conceptual, methodological, and theoretical issues. Mahwah (NJ): Lawrence Erlbaum Associates; 1998. p. 127–43.
[7] Moreland L. Somali Bantu refugees: cultural considerations for service providers. Bridging Refugee Youth and Children's Services Bulletin. Available at: http://www.brycs.org/documents/SBantu%20Service%20Considerations.pdf. Accessed December 4, 2007.
[8] Weine SM, Ware N, Lezic A. An ethnographic study of converting cultural capital in teen refugees and their families from Bosnia-Herzegovina. Psychiatr Serv 2004;55:923–7.

[9] Beiser M, Devins G, Dion R, et al. Immigration, acculturation and health. Report to the National Health Research and Development Program (NHRDP), Project No. 6606-6414-NPHS, Ottawa (Canada).

[10] Beiser M, Turner RJ, Ganesan S. Catastrophic stress and factors affecting its consequences among Southeast Asian refugees. Soc Sci Med 1989;28(3):183–95.

[11] Melville MB, Lykes MB. Guatemalan Indian children and the sociocultural effects of government-sponsored terrorism. Soc Sci Med 1992;34(5):533–48.

[12] Servan-Schreiber D, Lin BL, Birmaher B. Prevalence of posttraumatic stress disorder and major depressive disorder in Tibetan refugee children. J Am Acad Child Adolesc Psychiatry 1998;37:874–9.

[13] Simich L, Beiser M, Mawani FN. Social support and the significance of shared experience in refugee migration and resettlement. West J Nurs Res 2003;25(7):872–91.

[14] Fuligni AJ. The academic achievement of adolescents from immigrant families: the role of family background, attitudes, and behavior. Child Dev 1997;68:261–73.

[15] Suarez-Orozco C, Suarez-Orozco M. Children of immigration. Cambridge (MA): Harvard University Press; 2001.

[16] Birman D, Trickett EJ, Vinokurov A. Acculturation and adaptation of Soviet Jewish refugee adolescents: predictors of adjustment across life domains. Am J Community Psychol 2002; 30:585–607.

[17] Fiese BH, Sameroff AJ, Grotevant HD, et al. Observing families through the stories they tell: a multidimensional approach. In: Kerig P, Lindahl K, editors. Family observational coding systems: resources for systemic research. Mahwah (NJ): LEA; 2001. p. 259–72.

[18] Weine SM, Feetham S, Kulauzovic Y, et al. A multiple-family group access intervention for refugee families with PTSD. J Marital Fam Ther 2008;34:149–64.

[19] Weine SM, Kulauzovic Y, Besic S, et al. A family beliefs framework for developing socially and culturally specific preventive interventions for refugee families and adolescents. Am J Orthopsychiatry 2006;76:1–9.

[20] Weine SM, Raijna D, Kulauzovic Y, et al. The TAFES multi-family group intervention for Kosovar refugees: a descriptive study. J Nerv Ment Dis 2003;191(2):100–7.

[21] Szapocznik J, Santisteban D, Kurtines W, et al. Bicultural effectiveness training: a treatment intervention for enhancing intercultural adjustment in Cuban American families. Hisp J Behav Sci 1984;6(4):317–44.

[22] Family Strengthening Policy Center. Introduction to family strengthening. Policy brief No. 1. Available at: http://www.nassembly.org/fspc/practice/documents/Brief1.pdf. Accessed December 4, 2007.

[23] United States Conference of Catholic Bishops. Strengthening refugee families and marriages. Available at: http://www.usccb.org/mrs/mfs.shtml. Accessed December 4, 2007.

[24] Office of Refugee Resettlement. Achievement and Challenge Proceedings: 2004 National Refugee Program Consultation. Washington, DC: Administration for Children and Families, US Department of Health and Human Services; June 23–25, 2004.

[25] Williams CL. Prevention programs for refugees: an interface for mental health and public health. J Prim Prev 1989;10:167–86.

[26] Williams CL. Toward the development of preventive interventions for youth traumatized by war and refugee flight. In: Apfel RJ, Simon B, editors. Minefield in their hearts: the mental health of children in war and communal violence. New Haven (CT): Yale University Press; 1996. p. 201–17.

[27] Litz BT, Gray MJ, Bryant RA, et al. Early intervention for trauma: current status and future directions. Clinical Psychology: Science and Practice 2002;9(2):112–34.

[28] World Health Organization in collaboration with the Prevention Research Centre of the Universities of Nijmegen and Maastricht. Prevention of mental disorders: effective interventions and policy options: summary report. Geneva (Switzerland): World Health Organization; 2004.

[29] Mrazek PJ, Haggerty RJ, editors. Reducing risks for mental disorders: frontiers for preventive intervention research. Washington, DC: National Academy Press; 1994.

[30] Amodeo M, Peou S, Grigg-Saito D, et al. Providing culturally specific substance abuse services in refugee and immigrant communities: lessons from a Cambodian treatment and demonstration project. Journal of Social Work Practice and Addiction 2004;4(3):23–46.

[31] Berman H. Children and war: current understandings and future directions. Public Health Nurs 2001;18:243–52.

[32] Yule W. From pogroms to "ethnic cleansing": meeting the needs of war affected children. J Child Psychol Psychiatry 2000;41(6):695–702.

[33] Yang K. Southeast Asian American children: not the "model minority". In children of immigrant families. Future Child 2004;14(2):127–33.

[34] Miller KE. Beyond the front stage: trust access and the relational context in research with refugee communities. Am J Community Psychol 2004;33(3–4):217–27.

[35] Lustig S, Kia-Keating M, Knight W, et al. Review of child and adolescent refugee mental health. J Am Acad Child Adolesc Psychiatry 2004;43(1):24–36.

[36] US Committee for Refugees. Cry for help: Refugee menaqtal health in the United States. Refugee Reports 1997;18(9):1–7.

[37] Fox SH, Tang SS. The Sierra Leonean refugee experience: traumatic events and psychiatric sequel. J Nerv Ment Dis 2000;188(8):490–5.

[38] Watters C. Emerging paradigms in the mental health care of refugees. Soc Sci Med 2001; 52(11):1709–18.

[39] Szapocznik J, Coatsworth JD. An ecodevelopmental framework for organizing risk and protection for drug abuse: a developmental model of risk and protection. In: Glantz M, Hartel CR, editors. Drug abuse: origins and interventions. Washington, DC: American Psychological Association; 1999. p. 331–66.

[40] Szapocznik J, Kurtines W, Santisteban DA, et al. The evolution structural ecosystemic theory for working with Latino families. In: Garcia J, Zea MC, editors. Psychological interventions and research with Latino populations. Boston: Allyn, Bacon, Publishers; 1997. p. 166–90.

[41] Garmezy N. Vulnerability research and the issue of primary prevention. Am J Orthopsychiatry 1971;41(1):101–16.

[42] Beardslee WR, Gladstone TR. Prevention of childhood depression: recent findings and future prospects. Biol Psychiatry 2001;49(12):1101–10.

[43] Beardslee WR, Gladstone TRG, Wright EJ, et al. A family-based approach to the prevention of depressive symptoms in children at risk: evidence of parental and child change. Pediatrics 2003;112(2):119–31.

[44] Substance Abuse Mental Health Services Administration. Science-based prevention programs and principles: effective substance abuse and mental health programs for every community. Rockville (MD): US Department of Health and Human Services; 2002.

[45] Rutter M. Psychosocial adversity: risk, resilience and recovery. Southern African Journal of Child and Adolescent Psychiatry 1995;7(2):75–88.

[46] Silverman M. Children of psychiatrically ill parents: a prevention perspective. Hosp Community Psychiatry 1989;40(12):1257–64.

[47] Werner EE. Overcoming the odds. J Dev Behav Pediatr 1994;15(2):131–6.

[48] Werner EE. High-risk children in young adulthood: a longitudinal study from birth to 32 years. Am J Orthopsychiatry 1989;59(1):72–81.

[49] Kumpfer KL, Alvarado R. Strengthening families to prevent drug use in multi-ethnic youth. In: Botvin G, Schinke S, Orlandi M, editors. Drug abuse prevention with multi-ethnic youth. Newbury Park (CA): Sage Publications; 1995. p. 253–94.

[50] Luthar SS, Zigler E. Vulnerability and competence: a review of research on resilience in childhood. Am J Orthopsychiatry 1991;61(1):6–22.

[51] Fan X, Chen M. Parental involvement and student's academic achievement: a meta-analysis. Educational Psychology Review 2001;13(1):1–22.

[52] Timm JT. Hmong values and American education. Equity & Excellent in Education 1994; 27(2):284–8.

[53] Smith-Hefner NJ. Language and identity in the education of Boston-area Khmer. Anthropol Educ Q 1990;21:250–68.

[54] Simon R. Refugee families' adjustment and aspirations: a comparison of Soviet Jewish and Vietnamese immigrants. Ethn Racial Stud 1983;6(4):492–504.

[55] Family Strengthening Policy Center. Parental involvement in education. Policy brief No. 3. Available at: http://www.nassembly.org/fspc/practice/documents/Brief3.pdf. Accessed December 4, 2007.

[56] Henderson AT, Mapp KL. A new wave of evidence: the impact of family, school, community connections on student achievement. Austin (TX): Southwest Educational Development Laboratory; 2002.

[57] Kia-Keating M, Ellis BH. Belonging and connection to school in resettlement: young refugees, school belonging, and psychosocial adjustment. Clin Child Psychol Psychiatry 2007;12(1):29–43.

[58] McBrien JL. Educational needs and barriers for refugee students in the United States: a review of the literature. Rev Educ Res 2005;75(3):329–64.

[59] The Right Question Project. Available at: www.rightquestion.org. Accessed December 4, 2007.

[60] Parent Institute for Quality Education. Available at: www.piqe.org. Accessed December 4, 2007.

[61] McKay M, Paikoff R, Baptiste D, et al, CHAMP Collaborative Board. Family-level impact of the CHAMP Family Program: a community collaborative effort to support urban families and reduce youth HIV risk exposure. Fam Process 2004;43(1):77–91.

[62] Epstien J, Dauber S. School programs and teacher practices of parent involvement in inner-city elementary and middle schools. The Elementary School Journal 1991;91(3):289–305.

[63] Rapkin BD, Tricket EJ. Comprehensive dynamic trial designs for behavioral prevention research with communities: overcoming inadequacies of the randomized controlled trial paradigm. In: Trickett E, Pequegnaut W, editors. Increasing the community impact of HIV preventive interventions. New York: Oxford University Press; 2005. p. 249–77.

[64] Weine SM, Knafl K, Feetham S, et al. A mixed-methods study of refugee families engaging in multi-family groups. Fam Relat 2005;54:558–68.

ELSEVIER
SAUNDERS

Child Adolesc Psychiatric Clin N Am
17 (2008) 533–549

CHILD AND
ADOLESCENT
PSYCHIATRIC CLINICS
OF NORTH AMERICA

School-Based Prevention Programs for Refugee Children

Cécile Rousseau, MD, MSc*, Jaswant Guzder, MD

Department of Psychiatry, McGill University, 7085 Hutchison,
Room 204.2, Montreal, Quebec, Canada H3N 1Y9

Global migratory phenomena are shaping the experiences of families flee-ing war, dictatorships, or poverty and insecurity linked to social turmoil. Al-though survival and the absence of meaningful prospects for the future, for oneself or one's family, still are very powerful incentives for migration, the chances of obtaining asylum have declined progressively as international mi-gration control policies have become a burning issue in Western countries. In this context, the number of accepted refugees and asylum seekers has been falling, and that of undocumented immigrants and those who have an uncertain, precarious status has been rising. Simultaneously, immigration to North America has shifted from a majority of European immigrants to a majority of immigrants from developing countries, including large num-bers of families fleeing direct persecution or social insecurity in their country of origin, thus blurring the classical distinction between immigrant and ref-ugee [1]. As a result, many immigrant and refugee children share a common direct or family experience of organized violence in their homeland and a context of poverty combined with a precarious social environment in the host country [2–4]. Despite this high exposure to adversity, immigrant and refugee families persistently underutilize mental health services [5,6]. Therefore schools play a key role, both as mediators in helping children and youths adapt to their host country and as the main access point to pre-vention and treatment services for mental health problems.

Even if the theoretic importance of schools is well recognized, educa-tional institutions, like other host-country institutions, often unwittingly replicate minority–majority tensions and become places where exclusion and discrimination are experienced at different levels by immigrant and ref-ugee children [7,8]. For children who have identified difficulties, cultural

* Corresponding author.

E-mail address: cecile.rousseau@mcgill.ca (C. Rousseau).

1056-4993/08/$ - see front matter © 2008 Elsevier Inc. All rights reserved.
doi:10.1016/j.chc.2008.02.002
childpsych.theclinics.com

misunderstandings about mental health or educational issues may produce problems regarding diagnosis and the appropriateness of the treatment and remedial measures proposed [9]. For example, mental health intervention may accelerate marginalization by labeling adjustment problems stemming from migratory difficulties or resistance strategies adopted by adolescents to respond to social inequalities as behavioral disorders [10,11].

In countries hosting a large number of immigrant and refugee children, schools are the institutions best positioned to implement prevention and treatment programs [12,13]. Tolfree [14] suggests a number of ways in which schools can meet the psychosocial needs of children affected by war or displacement, especially through programs that provide them with avenues for emotional expression, personal support, and opportunities to enhance their understanding of their past experiences. Setting up a classroom program to prevent psychologic distress in newly arrived immigrant and refugee children presents several challenges, however. First, the population is heterogeneous, both culturally and in terms of experiences in their homeland and during migration. Furthermore, the gap between school and family is wide, and a program devised by host-country therapists or educators easily could become just one more disparate element in the children's two separate worlds [15]. Last, despite many small-scale innovative projects, little is known, either in theory or in practice, about the types of activity that may work best for children from different cultural backgrounds [16]. In spite of these difficulties, numerous school programs, often based on ecologic principles, have been developed to prevent emotional and behavioral problems and to foster the ability of adolescent refugees to adapt to their new lives [14].

This article reviews the school programs developed to improve the mental health of refugee children, available through initiatives or activities integrated into the curriculum or for specific groups identified as being at risk or through mental health services located within the school. These programs address a wide range of issues but focus on overall adaptation and well-being and place special emphasis on the psychologic consequences of trauma or loss.

First, the authors briefly review the role of school-based prevention programs in the area of youth mental health and define prevention for refugee children. Second, they present programs that seek to facilitate the overall adjustment of refugee children to the host country through a transformation of the school environment and curriculum and then look at programs that use a specific treatment modality (creative expression or spirituality) or that focus on a specific issue (intercommunity tensions). Third, they describe some of the secondary prevention programs that have been proposed to overcome the underutilization of services through the implementation of school-based mental health services. For each type of program, they review the existing literature produced by nongovernmental organizations or schools working in the field, briefly discuss the existing evaluations and any related evidence, and illustrate the different categories of intervention by describing some representative programs.

Prevention programs for refugee children: between standard practice and cultural specificity

In the field of refugee studies, posttraumatic stress disorder (PTSD) seems to be the most popular descriptor of refugee illness and distress [17]. As a result, programs addressing PTSD are the most common and are given top priority. Recently, however, longitudinal studies of outcomes and meta-analyses of risk and protection factors for refugees have emphasized the importance of postmigration social factors [18], suggesting that greater consideration of the social environment may required within prevention and treatment programs and policies. In an analysis of European Union good practices in refugee health, Watters and Ingleby [19] stress the risk inherent in a victimizing perspective that portrays refugees as passive, helpless, and afflicted by psychopathology and insist on the need to co-construct services and programs with the refugees themselves to develop culturally appropriate interventions and to foster a sense of ownership and empowerment in refugee communities. These authors put the emphasis on school-based preventive activities for refugee youth, arguing that school-based prevention programs and activities should represent an alternative to current mental health practices. In a paper on prevention for refugee children, Williams [20] notes that prevention is difficult to define when speaking about refugee mental health because the notions of prevention and promotion have been borrowed from the public health field and cannot be transferred to directly mental health. In mental health, prevention may be used both in the context of diagnosable illnesses and to address the psychologic distress or interpersonal turmoil that may stem from adverse life experiences. Williams distinguishes among three types of prevention: primary, which is directed toward a group before significant maladjustment is experienced; secondary, which enables a person to regain his or her normal level of function and prevents further development of illness after its occurrence; and tertiary, which focuses on rehabilitation and on limiting the impairment associated with an illness.

At present, school-based prevention programs for refugee children are being developed at a time when evidence-based studies are guiding mainstream professional practices. In a review of the evidence supporting 322 evaluative studies of school programs, Green and colleagues [21] underscore the frequent lack of grounding in theory of the diverse interventions proposed and the absence of careful evaluation of many potentially interesting initiatives. In that review, culture and the migratory or refugee context are not mentioned. Increasingly, program designs must refer in some way to the practice parameters defining the reference standard in a particular field. The

American Association of Child and Adolescent Psychiatry (AACAP) PTSD practice parameters for children and adolescents [22] state that in trauma-related situations, the most commonly recommended interventions are focused on trauma and include some degree of direct discussion of it. Cognitive behavior therapy is at the forefront of evaluated techniques, as are some relaxation techniques. Some school-based grief- and trauma-focused psycho-therapy methods are mentioned also, including the intervention performed and evaluated by Goenjian and colleagues [23] in Armenian schools after an earthquake. Similarly, in the AACAP practice parameters for psychiatric consultation in schools [24], although the main emphasis is on clinical consultation, school-based prevention programs that have been found to be effective for children presenting some symptoms without reaching full diagnostic criteria are recommended in the aftermath of traumatic exposure [25–27]. These recommendations include a very broad statement about the need to consider the local cultural and social characteristics in the school consultation process.

Within the practice parameters the understandable concern for rigor, replicability, and evidence may favor the development of preventive intervention programs for minority, refugee, and immigrant children that tend to replicate programs developed for mainstream North American children without giving sufficient consideration to refugee-specific characteristics. This practice, in turn, may compromise the validity of the intervention and the measurement instrument used to assess its efficacy [28]. In this context, one of the risks of standardization is that it leaves no room for the integration of community voices and knowledge or the development of alternatives to mainstream approaches [19,20]. On the other hand, because of the precariousness of refugee family situations and the wide heterogeneity of refugee children, many innovative initiatives rooted in school and refugee community experiences have not been evaluated in a way that facilitates transferability.

Programs that address the overall adaptation of refugee children to host-society schools

A number of school programs try to avoid medicalizing the problems of refugee children and raising the potential stigma of being considered "at risk." These programs are directed at broader aspects of the social experience of these children and their families rather than at discrete psycho-pathologic manifestations. These programs target three main areas: the adjustment of the school to the needs of refugee children through professional development, the improvement of the relationship between the school and the home, and the development of classroom or after-school programs intended for the children themselves.

Many programs have a teacher-training and teacher-support component, especially at the elementary level where children have a more direct, ongoing relationship with a specific teacher. Although some teachers become passionate advocates of refugee children and may work outside their academic role to support refugee families, others are quite reluctant to take refugee-specific characteristics into consideration. This reluctance needs to be understood. On the one hand, teachers may fear being overwhelmed by the complexity of the situation and by their own limitations in trying to deal with it. On the other hand, contact with the refugee experience may force teachers to face the reality of human rights abuses in their immediate environment, a confrontation that may elicit anxiety and feelings of insecurity. Different methods have been proposed to support and train teachers. For example, in a London borough, refugee support teachers have a mandate to provide peer support, including supervision of classroom management and case discussion and also counseling for feelings of helplessness and anger aroused by empathy with the situation of refugee families in the host country [13]. Other schools emphasize cultural competency training for teachers or professional development courses that examine refugee mental health issues [29]. Although teacher training is a component of most initiatives, some qualitative evaluations of classroom programs note that the intervention per se often also constitutes an eye-opener for the teachers, who suddenly see their students and their families in another light [30].

The home–school relationship is another challenging area. The literature on family–school interactions focuses on the quality of the relationship over time and on the importance of reaching a shared understanding of situations [31,32]. From this perspective, the involvement of parents is conceptualized as an empowerment process through concrete practices [33]. This emphasis on empowerment is particularly appropriate because of the striking power imbalance between refugee families and host-country institutions. Beyond common obstacles of interpretation and translation caused by the language barrier, creating family–school links is a difficult task because of diverging perceptions about the role of the school and the participation of parents and about the definition of "normal" child development [34,35]. Quite often, North American schools promote autonomy as a key value, whereas immigrant and refugee families stress the importance of conforming to family or community norms [36]. Frequently, community organizations play a key role as mediators among students, their families, and the school, especially when feelings of distrust are present on all sides [37].

In the last few decades some very promising classroom programs have been developed specifically for refugee children in the Netherlands. The Pharos school-based prevention program is based on the premise that school has healing capacities because it provides children with personal attention and structure while encouraging their socialization with peers and with meaningful adults in the host society. In this capacity, school serves as a bridge to the new society and allows refugee children to project themselves into the future. One of the basic principles of the Pharos program is that catering to children's problems and strengthening the support systems around them should occur simultaneously and can be implemented by teachers while performing their normal teaching duties [38].

The Pharos program provides activities in both elementary and high schools. For each developmental level, there is a training course for teachers supported by multimedia material, along with two series of classroom lessons focusing on the shared refugee experience and on recreating links at school and in the new social environment. Both elementary and high school programs rely on combined verbal and nonverbal techniques (eg, the creation of a personal book that brings together representations of family and home and representations of school through pictures, drawings, and stories). These activities cover a wide range of issues pertaining to the past and present (with a focus on daily life, school, and social relations). They also address identity issues, feelings of trust and safety, and developing a sense of agency.

The programs have been manualized and evaluated by youth and teachers in the Netherlands, although the results of the evaluation have not been published. Subsequently, the programs have been transferred to the United Kingdom and implemented in Kent and Manchester [19]. The transfer process highlighted the importance of contextual differences: in the United Kingdom, refugee children attend regular schools, whereas in the Netherlands they are segregated in special schools. In the United Kingdom, the prevailing multicultural model was no doubt a major factor in favor of involving refugee parents and the communities themselves in the running of the programs; in the Netherlands, the likelihood that most asylum-seeking families would to be deported at some point considerably limited their interest in learning Dutch and consequently their link to the schools. This small-scale transfer experiment shows that the sociopolitical context of the refugee-receiving country is a crucial consideration in shaping the prevention program and that more attention should be given to the localization and empowerment of programs than to content standardization.

Programs that use a specific treatment modality: artistic expression as a means of promoting child mental health

Play and artistic expression are used commonly in therapeutic and educational settings. Improved self-esteem, expression of emotions, problem solving, and conflict resolution are the most frequently mentioned benefits of therapy methods based on creative expression [39,40]. Although creative expression frequently is used clinically and in groups of children at risk, few programs have undergone impact assessment. In the last 20 or 30 years, creative expression activities have come to be regarded as a good way of working with migrant children, helping them construct meaning and identity [41,42], and with refugee children or others who have experienced armed conflict [43], allowing them to work through their losses, come to terms with trauma, and re-establish social ties broken by repression [15,39–43].

With a view to building on prior work documenting the usefulness of creative expression programs for immigrant and refugee children in clinical and community settings [15,43–46], a Montreal team made up of schools, community organizations, and health professionals developed a set of prevention programs for preschools, elementary schools, and high schools. The aim of the programs was to help recently arrived children and adolescents bridge the gaps between home and school and between past and present and to work through experiences of loss and trauma [44–48].

Designed for preschoolers, the sandplay program consists of 10 workshops, given every second week over a period of 4 months, which are integrated into the regular kindergarten school day. As the opening ritual for each session, the children sit in a circle to sing an action song. They then create their own worlds in sand trays. The class is divided into groups of four. In the sand trays, the children have the opportunity to play by themselves or with the other children in their group, using verbal and nonverbal expression. They can choose from a variety of traditional sandplay figurines: people, animals, vehicles, housing, food, religious figures, and so on. The results of an earlier pilot project had shown, however, that a relative lack of multicultural figurines limited the children's ability to create other-than-host-society scenes, so the authors added a number of culturally diverse spiritual symbols and everyday figurines: different types of housing, people in national costumes, flags of different countries, and houses of worship and deities of several religions. Sometimes a theme is suggested, which the children may explore if they wish. The themes suggested are related to the children's everyday lives: for example, family, siblings, transportation to school, language, seasons. After creating a world, the children are invited to share with their group the story of the scenes they have created, supported by an adult from the intervention team. The closing ritual is another action song led by the teacher [47].

The elementary creative workshop program is made up of three types of activities and always combines verbal and nonverbal means of expression (drawing or painting a picture and telling or writing a story); during the activities the children alternate between working on their own and going back to their groups to listen or to present their work. In the first activity, children illustrate and comment on myths, tales, or legends from nondominant cultures. These stories are used to represent the stress and tension but also the richness of a minority position, although the traditions to which they refer are not necessarily those of the participating children. The stories are chosen to evoke specific themes to do with migration or the transformation induced by traumatic experiences. Qualitative analysis of the children's productions showed that myths of the homeland provide a basic framework on which to build a representation of experience and emotions [48]. Myths facilitate the attribution of meaning to a personal or family experience of trauma or migration [49]. They propose a narrative structure, a set of shared symbols and coping strategies, and a specific vision of time [50]. Having been handed down from generation to generation, they provide a reassuring structure, but they are malleable and flexible enough to be appropriated and adapted. Thus the workshop stories become adaptable metaphors that children can use to structure their own experiences. In the second activity, called "The Trip," the children are asked to draw and tell the story of a character of their choice who has been through a migration process. They are encouraged to tell or draw about the past (life in the homeland before migration), the trip itself, the arrival in the host country, and the future. In the last activity, the "Memory Patchwork," the children are asked to bring in myths and tales from their families and communities; these provide a more direct representation of the children's identities [51]. Children usually bring in one of three types of stories: traditional tales, historical accounts, or stories about family experiences. This activity reinforces the dialogue between children and their parents about positive aspects of their past and helps bridge the gap between home and school by symbolically introducing the family into the classroom.

Finally, the high school program is based on Boal's forum and Fox's playback theater. Playback theater is a type of improvisational theater that aims to achieve personal and social transformation through sharing a theater experience within a ritual space [52]. It places the marginalized and excluded in the position of subject, which can empower them to change themselves and their environment [53,54]. The drama program was developed in a multiethnic district in Montreal with a high proportion of recently arrived immigrants and refugees. The goal of the drama therapy program was to give young immigrants and refugees a chance to reappropriate and share group stories, to help them construct meaning and identity in their personal stories and establish a bridge between the past and the present. The workshop is part of the regular school day. The teachers are present and participate whenever they wish to, for example by commenting or contributing a personal story. The students take part in 12 weekly sessions. Within a safe and respectful atmosphere, a play director supports the storyteller by eliciting the story as it unfolds, while actors and musicians gather the information to play the story back to the teller and the group. The stories told can be transformed and replayed through alternative scenarios developed by the group of adolescents. The idea is to alter the situation to empower the storyteller and the others, by changing the meaning, building a relationship, or creating an opening or dialogue with others that was missing from the original story. This part of the workshop becomes a collective effort, focusing on co-creating a story or situation in which the adolescents look for alternatives to their first reactions and strategies. Supported by the intervention team, the young people use sound, movement, and a few words while relying mostly on images and working with metaphor to reflect the point of view and feelings of the teller.

Repeated qualitative evaluations identified four key elements indicative of the effects of the workshops: constructing a safe space, acknowledging and valuing multiplicity, establishing continuity, and transforming adversity [55]. A quantitative evaluation (experimental versus control) of the three programs (preschool, elementary, and high school) showed that all had a significant effect on child and youth mental health. At the elementary level they increased children's self-esteem and reduced their level of emotional and behavioral symptoms [30]. In high school they diminished impairment and improved school performance [56]. Finally, in preschool, the evaluation took place just after the tsunami, and results provided evidence that the creative workshops can have a beneficial effect on preschoolers who have experienced adversity either directly or through intergenerational transmission and also may provide some protection against a retriggering of trauma in such children when exposed to distressing events through the media, as occurred with the tsunami [48].

Despite follow-up requests from the schools, replication of these successful and innovative programs has been limited by the lack of resources needed to implement them in their current format. At present, teachers and specialized resources in schools, who always have been an essential part of the team, are being trained to reproduce the workshops without the on-site support of the external research team, thus reducing the cost of the programs and making it possible to implement them on a broader scale.

Programs inspired by tradition and spirituality

Traumatic experiences often challenge the belief systems of individuals, families, and communities. Religious and spiritual belief can be either shattered or strengthened as people struggle to make sense of their experiences. Spirituality often occupies an important place in healing and may even intervene in the clinical realm, either through a quest for meaning or as an integral part of the reconstruction process [57]. For refugee children, religion and spirituality may provide tools to mourn the diverse losses they or their families have undergone and also may help them make sense of a world in which evil may be too present and in which parental figures may seem helpless to provide needed protection. Although no school-based prevention programs have focused directly on spirituality as a means of fostering resiliency, some community organizations provide interesting examples of how traditional rituals may play a preventive role [20].

Duncan and Kang (unpublished manuscript, 1985) describe a program targeting unaccompanied Cambodian minors resettled by Catholic community services in Tacoma, Washington. Theravada Buddhist ceremonies and rituals to honor the dead and consultation with Buddhist spiritual leaders were among the main components of the program designed to help these young people overcome the staggering losses they had suffered. Three ceremonies were performed for each of the unaccompanied minors and their foster families during the first year of the resettlement. The qualitative evaluation suggested that the program promoted grief resolution, reduced sleep disturbance and spirit visits, and increased foster family bonding. Although it clearly is not the mandate of the school to enter into the religious realm, it may be worthwhile for schools to establish links with religious and spiritual leaders who support refugee communities. Such leaders may provide bridging and networking for more isolated families, who may express spiritual longing or the need to reconnect to a religious group.

Moral development programs: the challenge of the awareness of the other in a polarized global world

The current international situation is characterized by mounting intercommunity tensions, a widespread culture of fear, and a striking reduction in opportunities for dialogue and willingness to debate [58,59]. The oversimplification of the representation of the "other" directly influences the way in which majority and minority children perceive themselves and their peers. Conflict-situation research suggests that children's moral development and mental health are linked and underscores the temporary protective effect of a strong ideology portraying the collective self as good and the enemy as evil, although this position actually may fuel the conflict and hamper reconciliation [60]. Greater long-term resiliency may be associated with the capacity to perceive complexity, face moral dilemmas, and develop empathy and awareness of the other [61]. In multiethnic societies the latter position ultimately may be more protective because it can help children resolve the loyalty conflict between school and home.

Schools are at the forefront in the transmission of representations (stereotypical or not) of the "other." In this capacity, they have been used less to promote conflict resolution than to increase partisanship and further aggravate conflicts by radicalizing children and recruiting them [62]. Although diverse conflict-resolution models have been proposed—antiracist pedagogy, peace education, conflict resolution approaches [63]—very few programs have addressed the ways in which these programs should be adapted in multiethnic societies that must integrate refugee and immigrant children.

During the Iraq war, a school-based preventive pilot project was developed to reduce anxiety and intergroup tensions in recent immigrant refugee children [64]. The project was structured to take advantage of the school's key position as the meeting point between the world of the homeland and home and the world of the host country. Its principal aim was to create a space—a political forum—that would allow peaceful and respectful coexistence of these different worlds, without pushing for consensus or convergence.

Different activities were organized. Children were asked to bring in newspaper clippings or short summaries of television or radio programs that interested them. Because not all children had access to newspapers, some newspapers were also provided by the school. To ensure representation of a range of viewpoints and identities, children were encouraged to bring in papers in different languages (mainly French, English, Urdu, and Hindi). Children worked in groups to decide which news stories or issues would be discussed. Decisions about a general topic or specific activity (drawing, writing a letter together) were taken collectively. The children usually wanted to vote and abided by the results of the votes.

In the forum, the children were able to go back and forth naturally between discussing highly charged issues and joking or chatting about lighter topics. In that sense, the forums provided the opportunity to identify with the traumatic experiences of other communities while simultaneously maintaining a distance from painful emotions when they became too much to bear. The forum also made room for the respectful coexistence of a multiplicity of voices: the children's voices and the collective voices of a number of communities represented in the newspapers or stories discussed. The children were able to express empathy both for the families of the American soldiers who have died in Iraq and for the Iraqi families suffering from the bombing. The children felt a sense of agency when they decided to write a collective letter of solidarity calling for an end to the war, which they published in the school newspaper.

The analysis of the forum process and of the content brought in it by the children suggests that school may be a pivotal place where thinking about moral complexity can be taught in a way that counteracts the oversimplification and graphic images often channeled by the media. Transforming representations of the other and recognizing otherness in oneself may pave the way to a more peaceful future among minority and majority groups in our societies.

School-based mental health services

To address the underutilization of mental health services by immigrant children and certain minority groups, some initiatives aimed at providing clinical services through the school have been put forward. In this area, as in more adaptation-focused programs, the immigration context of the host country has a significant influence on what services are offered. A large number of Central American families fleeing war have taken refuge in the United States but have not been identified as refugees simply because they do not have this legal status. Some programs designed to respond generally to the needs of Latino children and families by improving the cultural sensitivity of the services they provide make a special effort to take into consideration the difficult migratory journey and premigratory trauma that many Central American families have experienced [65]. The AMIGO program, for instance, provides mental health services to 15 elementary schools in Montgomery County, Maryland. Its goals are to enhance students' personal, social, and academic development; to improve family communication and reduce stress; and to facilitate the cultural adjustments of recent arrivals to the host country [65]. The program offers a wide array of mental health services: individual, group, and family therapy; in-home and crisis intervention; school consultation; interagency collaboration; and parent education/ support. The emphasis is on building trust by catering to families' basic subsistence needs and facilitating access to services for those who cannot be reached by written material or telephone or who are unable to come to school.

AMIGO groups for children help them adjust to life in the United States, to cope with the grief and loss associated with premigratory adversity, to resolve language differences between home and school, and to promote multicultural appreciation. Although probably based on the subjective appraisal of parents, teachers, and the youths themselves, the program evaluation report states that AMIGO activities are perceived as bringing a significant improvement to the lives of the children and their families. A more in-depth qualitative and quantitative evaluation of the program would provide more objective support for these perceptions.

In California, a high level of exposure to violence was found in immigrant school children, with 49% of students reporting victimization in the previous year and 32% presenting with clinical levels of PTSD symptoms [4]. In response to these findings, the Los Angeles Unified School District developed a trauma-focused program called the Mental Health for Immigrant Program (MHIP). Although the MHIP was offered to a multiethnic group, most participants were Latino [25]. The intervention consisted of eight group sessions of cognitive behavioral therapy, and four 2-hour optional multifamily group sessions for parents, which included support for common experiences of loss and separation that many had suffered during migration.

The results of a quasi-experimental study conducted to evaluate the intervention showed a moderate decline in children's relative PTSD symptoms. According to the authors, these results suggest that cognitive behavioral therapy can be delivered effectively by school clinicians to treat children exposed to a wide range of community violence. The bias in participation may be related to the cultural appropriateness of group-based psychologic interventions, which may be more significant for some groups than for others [66].

The United Kingdom has been received a steady flow of refugee families, and clinical studies have suggested a high incidence of psychiatric disorders in these families [12]. To provide appropriate services for these children, a primary school in an inner London borough set up an on-site mental health unit to treat refugee children referred by their teachers [67]. Treatment chiefly addressed disorders related to past violence, losses, and present socioeconomic precariousness but also addressed specific learning and scholastic difficulties. Evaluation results showed a decline in overall symptom scores and highlighted the model's acceptability to children, families, and school. This small pilot project is the only published study about a school-based mental health service designed specifically for refugees. In all likelihood, the service was set up only because of the school's very high number of refugee children and strong advocacy position. Despite its limitations, the project underscores the difficulties inherent in providing mental health care to refugee children because of the persistent precariousness of their family and social environment, which forces the families into a survival mode that leaves them little time and energy for coming to terms with past adversity and adapting to the new society.

Summary

In light of the tendency of refugee families to underutilize mental health services and the high exposure of refugee children to adversity, there is a broad consensus that primary and secondary school-based prevention programs can play a key role in promoting the mental health of these children. Unfortunately, the development of school-based prevention programs is hindered by a number of major obstacles. First, refugee families and communities are afraid of the stigmatization that may be associated with any initiatives focusing on the adversity of their experiences, especially if these programs portray them as victims or use a psychopathologic model. Second, refugee children in schools represent a very heterogeneous group, both culturally and in terms of migratory experience, and it is not easy to address their diverse needs through culturally appropriate programs. Third, schools in refugee-receiving countries face widely different social and institutional realities; therefore the extensive local adaptations that are needed make program transferability challenging.

A review of existing school-based prevention program initiatives identifies a number of promising avenues:

- Ecologic models of intervention that address the whole-school environment are useful because they provide a systemic understanding of the interactions among the different players. They propose supporting and training teachers so that they can help their refugee students without becoming too distressed. These models also insist on parent–school interactions, which should be understood in terms of cultural differences and also as reflecting power imbalances between refugee families and host-country institutions.
- Classroom activities addressing the overall adjustment of refugee children to the host society and their well-being have an important role. They support the children in assimilating past and present experiences by presenting these as learning opportunities, facilitating emotional expression with respect to the experiences, and promoting the development of relationships among refugee children and with children and adults of the host society.

- Some prevention programs that use specific treatment modalities such as artistic expression also seem to be protective at different moments of children's development. They can be implemented in kindergarten, elementary school, or high school. They support the transformation of past and present adversity through creativity and metaphorical representations and foster the development of solidarity among children.
- Secondary prevention, which includes group intervention for children presenting with PTSD symptoms and school-based clinical services for individual children presenting with emotional and behavioral problems, seems to have some efficacy and to be well accepted by refugee parents. There is, however, a need to document more thoroughly the group or personal reluctances to participate in these services to understand better their cultural appropriateness.

In general, the development of school-based prevention programs seems to be hindered by three main factors. Health professionals' preoccupation with evidence-based treatment may hamper the already slow development of alternatives to mainstream practices, although these alternatives could provide a wider array of programs addressing the different cultural and contextual needs of refugee families. The existing services and programs developed by schools and nongovernmental community organizations often are not evaluated rigorously, either qualitatively or quantitatively. Finally, the precariousness of refugees' family and social environment hinders their capacity to become involved fully in the development of such programs.

Multidisciplinary school-based prevention programs that combine a mental health with an educational perspective and that promote a continuous partnership with community organizations may be one way of overcoming these obstacles.

References

[1] Rousseau C, Drapeau A. Premigration exposure to political violence among independent immigrants and its association with emotional distress. J Nerv Ment Dis 2004;192(12):852–6.
[2] Gurvitch A. What did we learn? A call to action to improve immigrants' access to mental health services. In: Danieli Y, Dingman RL, editors. On the ground after September 11: mental health responses and practical knowledge gained. New York: The Haworth Maltreatment and Trauma Press; 2005. p. 541–50.
[3] Beiser M, Hou F, Hyman I, et al. Poverty, family process, and the mental health of immigrant children in Canada. Am J Pub Health 2002;92(2):220–7.
[4] Jaycox LH, Stein BD, Kataoka SH, et al. Violence exposure, posttraumatic stress disorder, and depressive symptoms among recent immigrant schoolchildren. J Am Acad Child Adolesc Psychiatry 2002;41(9):1104–10.
[5] Laroche M. Health status and health services utilisation of Canada's immigrant and nonimmigrant populations. Can Public Policy 2000;26(1):51–73.
[6] Desmeules M, Gold J, Kazanjian A, et al. New approaches to immigrant health assessment. Can J Public Health 2004;95(3):122–6.

[7] Razack SH. Looking white people in the eye: gender, race and culture in courtrooms and classrooms. Toronto: University of Toronto Press; 1998 [incorporated (reprint 1999, 2001)].

[8] Baker C, Varma M, Tanaka C. Sticks and stones: racism as experienced by adolescents in New Brunswick. Can J Nurs Res 2001;33(3):87–105.

[9] Rousseau C, Drapeau A, Corin E. School performance and emotional problems in refugee children. Am J Orthopsychiatry 1996;66(2):239–51.

[10] Solomon P. Black resistance in high school: forging a separatist culture. Albany (NY): State University of New York Press; 1993.

[11] James C, Braithwaite K. The education of African Canadians: issues, contexts and expectations. In: Braithwaite KS, James CE, editors. Educating African Canadian. Toronto: James Lorimer & Company, Ltd.; 1996. p. 13–32.

[12] Hodes M. Psychologically distressed refugee children in the United Kingdom. Child Psychology & Psychiatry Review 2000;5(2):57–68.

[13] Bolloten B, Spafford T. Supporting refugee children in East London primary schools. In: Jones JRC, editor. Refugee education—mapping the field. Oakhill (UK): Trentham Books Limited; 1998. p. 107–23.

[14] Tolfree D. Restoring playfulness—different approaches to assisting children who are psychologically affected by war or displacement. Stockholm (Sweden): Rädda Barnen/ Save the Children Sweden; 1996.

[15] Miller KE, Billings DL. Playing to grow: a primary mental health intervention with Guatemalan refugee children. Am J Orthopsychiatry 1994;64(3):346–56.

[16] Williams CL, Berry JW. Primary prevention of acculturative stress among refugees: application of psychological theory and practice. Am Psychol 1991;46(6):632–41.

[17] Ahearn FLJ. Psychosocial wellness: methodological approaches to the study of refugees. In: Frederick LA Jr, editor. Psychosocial wellness of refugees: issues in qualitative and quantitative research. New York: Berghahn Books; 2000. p. 3–23.

[18] Porter M, Haslam N. Predisplacement and postdisplacement factors associated with mental health of refugees and internally displaced persons: a meta-analysis. JAMA 2005;294(5): 602–12.

[19] Watters C, Ingleby D. Locations of care: meeting the mental health and social care needs of refugees in Europe. Int J Law Psychiatry 2004;27:549–70.

[20] Williams CL. Toward the development of preventive intervention for youth traumatized by war and refugee flight. In: Ahearn FL Jr, Athey JL, editors. Refugee children: theory, research, and services. Baltimore (MD): Johns Hopkins University Press; 1991.

[21] Green J, Howes F, Waters E, et al. Promoting the social and emotional health of primary school-aged children: reviewing the evidence base for school-based interventions. International Journal of Mental Health Promotion 2005;7(3):30–6.

[22] AACAP Official Action. Practice parameters for the assessment and treatment of children and adolescents with schizophrenia. J Am Acad Child Adolesc Psychiatry 1997;36(10): 177S–92S.

[23] Goenjian A, Karayan I, Pynoos R, et al. Outcome of psychotherapy among early adolescents after trauma. Am J Psychiatry 1997;154(4):536–42.

[24] AACAP. Practice parameter for psychiatric consultation to schools. J Am Acad Child Adolesc Psychiatry 2005;44(10):1068–84.

[25] Kataoka SH, Stein BD, Jaycox LH, et al. A school-based mental health program for traumatized Latino immigrant children. J Am Acad Child Adolesc Psychiatry 2003;42(3): 311–8.

[26] Chemtob CM, Nakashima J, Carlson CG. Brief treatment for elementary school children with disaster-related posttraumatic stress disorder: a field study. J Clin Psychol 2002; 58(1):99–112.

[27] Stein BD, Jaycox LH, Kataoka SH, et al. A mental health intervention for schoolchildren exposed to violence: a randomized controlled trial. JAMA 2003;290(5):603–11.

[28] Hollifield M, Warner TD, Lian N, et al. Measuring trauma and health status in refugees. JAMA 2002;288(5):611–21.

[29] Sleeter CE. Preparing teachers for culturally diverse schools: research and the overwhelming presence of whiteness. Journal of Teacher Education 2001;52(2):94–106.

[30] Rousseau C, Drapeau A, Lacroix L, et al. Evaluation of a classroom program of creative expression workshops for refugee and immigrant children. J Child Psychol Psychiatry 2005;46(2):180–5.

[31] Pena DC. Parent involvement: influencing factors and implications. J Educ Res 2000;94(1): 42–54.

[32] Lynch E, Stein RC. Parent participation by ethnicity: a comparison of Hispanic, black, and Anglo families. Except Child 1987;54(2):105–11.

[33] Epstein JL. School, family and community partnerships. Boulder (CO): Westview; 2001.

[34] Okagaki L, Sternberg RJ. Parental beliefs and children's school performance. Child Dev 1993;64(1):36–56.

[35] Warner R. The views of Bangladeshi parents on the special school attended by their young children with severe learning difficulties. British Journal of Special Education 1999;26(4): 218–23.

[36] Valsiner J. Culture and the development of children's action: a theory of human development. 2nd edition. New York: John Wiley & Sons; 1997.

[37] Thomas E. Culture and schooling: building bridges between research, praxis and professionalism. New York: John Wiley & Sons; 2000.

[38] Ingleby D, Watters C. Refugee children at school: good practices in mental health and social care. Education and Health 2002;20(3):43–5.

[39] Torbert M. Follow me: a handbook of movement activities for children. Englewood Cliffs (NJ): Prentice-Hall; 1990.

[40] Schaefer C. The therapeutic powers of play. Northvale (NJ): Aronson; 1993.

[41] Elbedour S, Bastien DT, Center BA. Identity formation in the shadow of conflict: projective drawings by Palestinian and Israeli Arab children from the West Bank and Gaza. J Peace Res 1997;34(2):217–31.

[42] Howard GS. A narrative approach to thinking, cross-cultural psychology and psychotherapy. Am Psychol 1991;46:187–97.

[43] Danev M. Library project "step by step to recovery". In: Dokter D, editor. Art therapists, refugees and migrants: reaching across borders. London: Jessica Kingsley; 1998.

[44] Nylund BV, Legrand JC, Holtsberg P. The role of art in psychosocial care and protection for displaced children. Forced Migration Review 1999;6:16–9.

[45] Akhundov N. Psychosocial rehabilitation of IDP children: using theatre, art, music and sport. Forced Migration Review 1999;6:20–1.

[46] Lopez A, Saenz I. Nuestro origen, nuestro exilio: de niño a niño. Mexico: Comité del Distrito Federal de Ayuda a Refugiados Guatemaltecos; 1992.

[47] Lacroix L, Rousseau C, Gauthier M-F, et al. Immigrant and refugee preschoolers' sandplay representations of tsunami. The Arts in Psychotherapy 2007;34:99–113.

[48] Rousseau C, Heusch N. The trip: a creative expression project for refugee and immigrant children. Am J Art Ther 2000;17(1):31–40.

[49] De Plaen S, Moro MR, Pinon-Rousseau D, et al. L'enfant qui avait une mémoire de vieux. Un dispositif de soins à recréer pour chaque enfant de migrants. Prisme 1998;8(3):44–76.

[50] Bagilishya D. Mettre des mots sur sa douleur. Le mauvais sort de Nazaire, mineur non accompagné réfugié au Canada en provenance d'Afrique. Prisme 1999;28:72–85.

[51] Rousseau C, Lacroix L, Bagilishya D, et al. Working with myths: creative expression workshops for immigrant and refugee children in a school setting. Journal of the American Art Therapy Association 2003;20(1):3–10.

[52] Fox J. Playback theater: the community sees itself. In: Schattner G, Courtney R, editors. Drama in therapy. New York: Drama Book Specialists; 1981. p. 295–306.

[53] Freire P. Pedagogy of the oppressed. New York: Seabury Press; 1970.

[54] Boal A. Théâtre de l'opprimé. New York: Urizen Books; 1979.
[55] Rousseau C, Singh A, Lacroix L, et al. Creative expression workshops for immigrant and refugee children. J Am Acad Child Adolesc Psychiatry 2004;43(2):235–8.
[56] Rousseau C, Benoit M, Gauthier M-F, et al. Classroom drama therapy program for immigrant and refugee adolescents: a pilot study. Clin Child Psychol Psychiatry 2007; 12(3):451–65.
[57] Boehnlein JK. Religion and spirituality after trauma. In: Kirmayer LJ, Lemelson R, Barad M, editors. Understanding trauma: integrating biological, clinical, and cultural perspectives. New York: Cambridge University press; 2007. p. 259–74.
[58] Information Center about Asylum and Refugee in the UK. Media image, community impact. Report of a pilot research study. London: ICAR; 2004 [report No.: 0954702425].
[59] Hörnqvist M. The birth of public order policy. Institute of Race Relations 2004;46(1):30–52.
[60] Punamäki R-L. Can ideological commitment protect children's psychosocial well-being in situations of political violence? Child Dev 1996;67:55–69.
[61] Apfel RJ, Simon B. Mitigating discontents with children in war: an ongoing psychoanalytic inquiry. In: Suárez-Orozco MM, Robben ACGM, editors. Cultures under siege: collective violence and trauma. Cambridge: Cambridge University Press; 2000. p. 102–30.
[62] Sluzki CE. Seeding violence in the minds of children. Am J Orthopsychiatry 2002;72(1):3–4.
[63] Lin Q. Toward a caring-centered multicultural education within the social justice context. Education 2001;122(1):107–14.
[64] Rousseau C, Machouf A. A preventive pilot project addressing multiethnic tensions in the wake of Iraq war. Am J Orthopsychiatry 2005;75(4):466–74.
[65] Greenberg Garrison E, Roy IS, Azar V. Responding to the mental health needs of Latino children and families through school-based services. Clin Psychol Rev 1999;19(2):199–219.
[66] Fox PG, Rossetti J, Burns KR, et al. Southeast Asian refugee children: a school-based mental health intervention. Int J Psychiatr Nurs Res 2005;11(1):1227–36.
[67] O'Shea B, Hodes M, Down G, et al. A school-based mental health service for refugee children. Clin Child Psychol Psychiatry 2000;5(2):189–201.

ELSEVIER
SAUNDERS

Child Adolesc Psychiatric Clin N Am
17 (2008) 551–568

CHILD AND
ADOLESCENT
PSYCHIATRIC CLINICS
OF NORTH AMERICA

Addressing the Mother–Infant Relationship in Displaced Communities

D. Rezzoug, MD[a,b,*], T. Baubet, MD[a,b],
G. Broder, MD[a], O. Taïeb, MD, PhD[a],
M.R. Moro, MD, PhD[a,b]

[a]*Department of Child and Adolescent Psychiatry (Bobigny, France), University Paris 13, 125 Rue de Stalingrad, 93000 Bobigny, France*
[b]*Doctors Without Borders, 8 rue Saint Sabin, 75077 Paris, France*

France remains a potential asylum destination for refugees, although the number of refugees resettling in France has been decreasing for several years according to statistics provided by the Office Français de Protection des Réfugiés et des Apatrides (OFPRA). This reduction was already appreciable in 2005 but was even more marked in 2006, with a decrease of 33.6% in asylum applications [1]. Recent changes in governmental responsibility and in administrative procedures (such as decreases in the time allowed between arrival in France and filing a first application and in the time allowed for appeals) make the administrative procedures even more difficult for individuals arriving in a country whose cultural, social, and legal systems may be disorienting and unfamiliar.

Refugees used to come under the purview of the Ministry for Foreign Affairs, with input from international organizations at work in the field. Now they come under the purview of the Ministry of the Interior. The management of refugees by the ministry that also supervises the regulation of immigration has led to unfortunate confusions between refugees and immigrants. The system does indeed suggest that refugees are immigrants, like any others. Although immigrants may come to France for any number of social, economic, or political reasons, refugees leave their country of origin in response to specific pressures. The changes in strategy affect the way in which refugees are received and recognized politically and culturally and may be responsible in part for the decreasing numbers of refugees resettling in

---

* Corresponding author. Department of Child and Adolescent Psychiatry, 125 Rue de Stalingrad, 93000 Bobigny, France.
E-mail address: dalila.rezzoug@avc.aphp.fr (D. Rezzoug).

1056-4993/08/$ - see front matter © 2008 Elsevier Inc. All rights reserved.
doi:10.1016/j.chc.2008.02.008   *childpsych.theclinics.com*

France. These increasing barriers to resettlement are exacerbated by the fact that infants and young children are rarely taken into account in receiving procedures.

The authors' own encounters with refugees have led them to consider certain specific features of these populations. These specific characteristics relate to exposure to three interlinked factors: the existence of traumatic experiences, the cultural dimensions of refugee experiences and how they are expressed, and the migratory experience. The authors' more particular focus within this broad field is the impact of this experience on the needs of parents or of mothers on their own and on the needs of their infants, whether born before or following exile.

This work is based on the authors' experience in the humanitarian aid field with Médecins sans Frontières in contexts of war and chronic conflict [2,3] and on their own expertise in transcultural psychiatry [4–7].

The premigratory experience and the experience of exile

Most patients that the authors encounter have come to France after fleeing their country. In most cases, they have left everything behind and have had to adapt to the loss of their cultural cocoon, the familiar world that enveloped them before departure. For some, the act of fleeing their country also involves loss and death of loved ones; and in some cases grieving may be compromised when nothing is known of the circumstances of a death, or where there is no body and no grave. For many, families are no longer present to cope alongside them, as would have been the case in their original social contexts where they would have found the cohesion of the family and the group, the familiar networks of arbitration and rituals, and all the other elements that enable the construction of a collective awareness. Excluded from or unable to access the cultural strategies needed to cope with death, separation, and grieving, some in these populations will be fragile and vulnerable [8–12].

Arrival in the country of refuge often is described as a difficult and decisive moment. France, the country that drafted the declaration of human rights, is perceived as a destination where people at last will feel safe, finally protected by a legitimate status as political refugees. The process to achieve this recognition is arduous and uncertain, however, often ending in refusal by the OFPRA. This body is the only channel for legal resettlement of asylum seekers.

Despite being vulnerable, refugees are required to tell the story of their ordeals and may be faced with frank suspicion or disbelief [8]. Loneliness, the loss of their roots and the aforementioned cultural supports, and disillusionment may contribute to asylum seekers' entertaining feelings of having no future and to the onset of depression. Thus, in the authors' experience, symptomatic decompensation most frequently occurs after exile, sometime several months or years later. The strategies aimed at survival that have been deployed before and during their flight are no longer functional after arrival in the receiving country [13]. In this social and psychologic context, familial and relational challenges inherent in any family situation are exacerbated by migration and the traumas it produces [14,15]. Finally, the establishment and development of harmonious parent–infant interactions can be complicated by a situation in which so much has been lost and disrupted and in which the transmission of expected parental cues and values can be compromised.

Clinical aspects of trauma in the context of exile

The notion of trauma is difficult to implement when working with patients from a wide range of cultural backgrounds. The state of posttraumatic stress, which is a concept that appeared at the end of the 1970s, has been described in the classification of the American Psychiatric Association's *Diagnostic and Statistical Manual of Mental Disorders* since 1980 [16]. It is used widely around the world to characterize the clinical patterns of trauma. It is not, however, suited to describing all patients and in particular those coping with situations of war, imprisonment, torture, or genocide, because it does not account for the changes brought about in the individual's personality itself or for the cultural coding of psychopathologic manifestations [17]. For one thing, the seriousness of the traumas is exacerbated because they arise from interpersonal or collective violence that is deliberate and organized by other human beings [8]. In addition, the traumas frequently are multiple, repeated, long-standing, and unaddressed. In this context, observed clinical manifestations sometimes correspond to what the International Statistical Classification of Diseases and Related Health terms "enduring personality change after catastrophic experience," or, more often, to the profile of complex posttraumatic stress disorder (PTSD) described by Herman [18–20] and defined by a clinical profile, which the authors summarize as

- Chronic difficulty in regulating and controlling emotions, in moderating reactions of anger, or in engaging in sexual activity, which leads to self-harming, suicidal, impulsive, or risk-related behaviors
- Attentional and consciousness disorders with total or partial amnesia or transitory dissociative episodes (depersonalization, de-realization, and others)
- Somatic complaints (often the primary reason for consultation), including chronic pain, functional somatic disorders, conversion symptoms, and sexual disorders
- Chronic alteration of personality accompanied by feelings of guilt or shame in relation to what has been experienced and a difficulty in establishing or maintaining relationships with others because of an inability to trust people, sometimes with aggressive tendencies toward others

• Changes in the systems of meaning, despairing feelings, and the loss of certain beliefs

Trauma in infants and children

Environments of war and collective violence affect families as well as individuals. These families, rendered more vulnerable by loss, displacement, and separation, are no longer able to assume their protective and containing roles, a loss that affects children in particular. Parents and responsible adults may be overwhelmed by their own reactions of fright and numbness and by their own responses to traumatic stress. In children, who in the past have been wrongly viewed as being somehow protected from trauma by their immaturity and their ability to forget, severe posttraumatic disturbances are observed and are all the more serious because they affect the development and construction of the child's unfolding personality [21,22].

Freud [23,24] has defined the notion of the barrier protecting the Self and the pathologic process that arises when this barrier is breached, and she argues that the period of greatest vulnerability is from birth through early infancy. She describes the impact on children of parental reactions toward traumatic events (their ability to protect and contain, or conversely their state of panic). Thus in babies and infants, even if the notion of death has not been acquired, it is thought that an event can generate a trauma if it overwhelms the child's defense abilities when there is no adult to protect that child, when the adult is unable to do so, or when the child perceives that there is no adult able to do so. The impact of a potentially traumatic event depends on developmental and environmental factors [25,26], including the development of the sensory organs, on psychomotor development (the ability to move and flee if necessary), on language development (both receptive and expressive), and on the ability of those around the child to ensure the functions of containment and protection. For Bailly [27] the traumatic potential among infants bears a relationship with some form of damage to the developing "infantile social theories," which also could be called "life theories." These are the set of fundamental beliefs and rules that the child starts to construct in the very first months of life and which are social and psychologic corollaries to the development of the cognitive ability to think. Thus trauma-generating events in a child are thought to be related to the absence of the early objects of love or affection during frightening events (an absence that the child's theories did not foresee), to external sensorial chaos (cold, heat, noise, light), and to internal sensorial factors (pain, hunger, thirst). "Chaos" for the baby also can be the mother's state of terror or posttraumatic disorganization or dissociation.

Winnicott [28], with reference to the stage of absolute dependency before the formation of a cogent self, has described early states of harrowing primitive agony that can occur and lead to defense organization of a psychotic type. In certain adults he noted the fear of a breakdown, which he understood as the fear of this harrowing state of agony underpinning the organization of defenses; he argued that this sense of potential collapse already had been experienced, that the breakdown already had occurred, but at a time when the Self was unable to experience it or retain it as a memory. Winnicott [29,30] underlines the importance of parental protection against this sort of psychotic core and provided a model for understanding the possible long-term psychic consequences of the earliest traumas, even in infants who almost certainly will not "remember" the traumatic events.

Among manifestations that are characteristic of older children (incompletely described by PTSD) are reliving manifestations, especially in the form of nightmares. Children may stop wanting to play and remain sad and prostrate. States of alarm accompanied by gripping gestures, phobic avoidance, or regressive behaviors, nocturnal enuresis, and refusal to sleep alone or in the dark all signal the loss of basic security and lead to regression in development and autonomy. Inhibition of thought and withdrawal can hinder learning processes and cognitive development. In the longer term, personality disorders can set in alongside the loss of fundamental beliefs that structure children and society (parental protection, rules, limits). These alterations can affect the processes of socialization [22,31–33].

Finally, it is worth noting that bodily expression of the disturbances is frequent among children and may be the most prominent feature. Such somatic complaints may include skin disorders (alopecia, psoriasis), pains (headache, abdominal pain), or faintness.

Trauma and early interaction

Although this discussion focuses on parents, it includes other adults and primary caregivers who are important in the child's life. Parent–infant interaction in situations of psychologic trauma can be altered by the effects of the child's trauma on parental function, by the effects of the trauma on the parents themselves, and through the consequences of these effects on the child. Thus behavioral alterations in a traumatized infant (which may be manifested by avoidance, withdrawal, agitation, and/or excitability) can contribute to the establishment of dysfunctional interaction within the mother–infant dyad. Likewise, traumatized mothers who are reliving traumatic events or who become withdrawn may no longer be available for their infants. Under some circumstances, usually involving severe sexual aggression or rape, the infant may be the object of violent or death-related projections when he or she is identified with the aggressor (particularly when the child is born as a result of rape or is born following rape of the mother). In the field of humanitarian operations in contexts of war or chronic conflict, these traumas are confounded by severe cases of malnutrition that resist medical treatment, accompanied by maternal rejection [34–37]. In Kosovo the authors frequently observed cases of breath-holding spells, in particular when several members of a family had been subjected to trauma. This dramatic symptom, which leads to an appearance of death in the child, can become a veritable family symptom leading to collective reliving of life-threatening events. The expression "shared PTSD" has been suggested to describe situations in which the response from the parents to the trauma undergone by the child creates a complex system of interactions that sustains the disturbances in both partners in the interaction [38]. The concept of "relational PTSD," developed by Scheeringa and Zeanah [39], describes the co-occurrence of a situation of psychologic trauma in the child and in the adult caring for the child, in which the symptoms of one exacerbate the symptoms of the other. Although the parents may have been absent at the time of the traumatic event, these authors describe three relational patterns:

- Withdrawal/nonreceptiveness/unavailability: a situation that often is encountered when the parents themselves have previously experienced trauma
- Overprotection/constriction: the parents are overwhelmed by the fear of another trauma occurring and by guilt at having been unable to protect the child
- Reconstitution of the traumatic scene/exposure to danger: the child's trauma is constantly reactivated by questions or allusions; the child is placed in situations where new traumas can occur

Cultural aspects of trauma

The expression given to suffering and the posttraumatic symptoms depend on age but also on the individual's culture. In their practice, the authors define psychologic trauma as a shock that the subject did not expect, accompanied by fright or terror. For Freud, fright results from a danger for which the subject is unprepared, the surprise element being characteristic: it was not possible to anticipate the event. Lebigot [40] describes fright (terror) as "that moment when a person sees himself as dead, and when he freezes in the face of that vision." Thus the trauma breaks into the psyche, imprinting a nonrepresentable experience. This characteristic remains remarkably consistent across cultures.

Depending on the culture to which the subject belongs, terror or fright is described in different ways, and what is expected or unexpected is different; but the authors argue that in all cases the trauma entails a breach between the inside and the outside, with an accompanying numbness, daze, or stupor. Nathan [41] put particular emphasis on the bipolar phenomenon of breach and extraction that can be found in all the traditional models for disturbances related to fright, and on the fact that these models can be compared with our own psychoanalytic models of psychic trauma. For example, in the Maghreb of North Africa, khal'a constitutes an explicative model for fright or terror. It contains the notion of shock, surprise, and terror. The subject affected registers fright that will remain latent and that will be reactivated if there is a further shock, a new fear (the notion of a threatening foreign body). In classical Arabic, this term ("fright") relates to the notion of removal, of tearing something away, and to the separation of body and soul. The flight of the soul leads to vulnerability and possible attack; attack sometimes can be envisaged as an invisible being (*djinn*) that takes possession of the frightened person [42]. The Quechua Indians in South America use the term "*susto*" to represent fright. Here, again, fright or terror creates a wound or injury, and the soul leaves the body. Other less specific representations that may be associated with traumas can be observed in certain areas of the world: *calor* in Salvador or *ataques de nervios* in Latin America. Somatization is a frequent signifier of that bodily experience. These manifestations can be sequelae of a trauma or signal a reliving process within the body.

A certain number of authors, including the teams of Baubet and Moro [42] or of Rousseau and Drapeau in Canada [43], have wondered if there might not be cultural invariance in the expression of suffering in connection with a traumatic event. They suggest that the elements that should be considered as invariants do not relate to the way in which suffering is expressed (ie, the symptoms) but rather to the underlying psychic processes. They support the idea that the symptoms responding to trauma vary according to the cultural context, but the symptoms nevertheless identify psychic processes that are common across cultures. They describe three of these processes: fright/terror, a change in the way the world is apprehended, and metamorphosis [42]. These notions mainly concern the adult, and few elements relating to children have been described.

Among the children of migrants, the notion of "etiologic theories" is interesting. In transcultural psychiatry, these are functional cultural parameters, that is, processes that generate discourse (or narrative) around the child. These are narratives that give "meaning to the meaningless" [44], to the misfortune that strikes a family or a group. The narratives concern meaning and not cause. Hence these theories are, for the parents, a way of giving meaning to issues affecting a child, which is, in fact, a culturally coded method of coping as well as a way of engendering a community around the child and family through mutual comprehension. There frequently are etiologies that present children as unusual in some way (sorcerer children, ancestor children, cursed children, and so forth). These representations at once bear meaning and enable the child to find a place in the group to which he belongs. They also can entail threats toward the child [45,46]. In transcultural therapy, these representations are useful as ways of engaging with children and families [5].

Providing care and therapeutic strategies

Tailoring care delivery

Few young children who have witnessed or undergone violence are referred to mental health specialists. This is particularly true for babies and children of refugee families. In this case, the compounding of social

difficulties (lack of stability, poverty, social isolation) and psychologic distress in the parents (posttraumatic stress, depression) renders the identification of such families, and the delivery of appropriate care, all the more
uncertain. Patients come to the care system most often via social workers
in contact with asylum seekers or via maternity hospitals and mother and
infant primary care centers. Patients also may be referred to the authors'
team after a medical consultation.

The authors' system for providing mental health care is intended for individuals who have undergone extreme trauma in settings of war, organized
persecution, imprisonment, and torture. Because the suffering expressed by
these patients is often massive, and because it is generated by very extreme
circumstances—"inhuman treatment that is organized deliberately, in the
course of which the very foundations of humanity are shaken" [8]—the system developed is multifocal and tailored. In addition to the more classic
therapeutic consultations (mother–infant and individual), models based on
team groups also may be implemented.

After a brief description of the team group model that the authors have
developed, the following sections consider the therapeutic strategies for
mother–infant situations, illustrated with a clinical case.

The trauma team group

This team model was developed from experience acquired over some 20
years with refugee patients in a transcultural approach based on the notion
that psychoanalysis and anthropology can be complementary. This transcultural psychotherapy was established in France by Nathan [14] for the first
generation of migrants, and then by Moro [47] for the second, using the
methodological principles of Devereux [48]: in any therapeutic relationship,
there is at once psychic universality and cultural encoding. The team group,
composed of four or five experienced therapists, trainees, and researchers,
usually is centered on the individual, receiving a patient, a couple, a dyad,
a parent–child triad, or a family. For mothers, either during pregnancy or
afterwards, mother–infant therapy can be offered if necessary. When families are received into the team model, the work consists mainly in supporting
parenting in the situation of exile and in exploring the impact of the trauma
on each member of the family and on the family as a whole.

This specific organization provides lengthy consultations for patients on
a monthly basis. The team group model is formed around a main therapist,
several cotherapists from different origins and cultural backgrounds, and
usually an interpreter so that patients can use their mother tongue. The
main therapist is the patient's direct interlocutor, "filtering" dealings among
the protagonists (cotherapists, interpreter, and patient). The group enables
representations to be circulated and enables the patient to build alliances
via diffracted transfer, allowing the coexistence of good and bad objects
without this coexistence being a threatening experience. The fact that there
are several cotherapists makes it possible to reduce the effects of numbness

and daze linked to the trauma in the patient and also in the therapists. The main therapist conducts the consultation and orchestrates interventions by the cotherapists as he or she sees fit. The cotherapists, who always address the main therapist, suggest metaphors and narratives to symbolize what they understand of the patient's history. Thus the patient is "fed" with representations that can enable him or her to rehabilitate his or her own abilities for association and symbolization.

There are certain special indications for this team model:

- When patients have been through psychologic trauma or experiences that are difficult to elaborate in a two-way relationship, the dynamics of a relationship can prevent the telling of the narrative (eg, for fear of destroying the therapist or of becoming the object of persecution).
- When there is difficulty in talking about the patient's cultural environment in the two-way relationship, there may be heavy silences on the subject or cultural representations that are difficult to broach and analyze in a two-way exchange (eg, experiences of possession or witchcraft). In these cases the team group enables a transcultural approach to the trauma.
- When patients are extremely isolated, the group dimension is mobilized as a prop and support. The group can supply new symbolic resources, memories, and representations on subjects such as death and grieving rituals.

The team therapy model enables the therapeutic process to get underway in situations where individual therapy becomes paralyzed (eg, in the case of massive reliving processes that obstruct any elaboration). Here the "holding" function of the group can be seen, as well as its ability to enable the therapists to sustain the faculty for thought whatever arises. Because the group provides real metaphoric and symbolic "nourishment," patients gradually retrieve their narrative resources and mobilize cultural strategies that ceased to function in the context of the trauma or were rendered inefficient by the migration [49,50].

Therapeutic strategies for mothers and infants

The parent–infant therapeutic process consists in working directly with the child and working on family interactions. In the present context, it is the parents who are burdened with the trauma, and the system has to be adapted to this context. Indeed, the protective role of the parent when faced with the infant's distress needs to be sustained. It therefore is important to provide individual care for the affected parent using individual and team group systems. It is in this sense that the system is "tailored."

The work on interactions aims mainly at restoring the ability for reflective functioning in the mother or, more generally, in the child's attachment figure. For Fonagy [51,52], this functioning concerns the ability of the attachment figure to represent the mental state of his or her child. In his view, a traumatized parent loses this ability for reflective function and therefore is unable to identify the thoughts, emotions, and intuitions of the child. This inability leads to inappropriate responses on the parent's part in the interaction. Affective tuning is altered. Here, the task of the mother–infant therapy is to spot the moments of failure to adapt and to mediate the interconnection. Lebovici [53] has emphasized the active part played by infants and what this part arouses in the therapist via "metaphorizing empathy," in which "it is the words that say what the body has felt in a moment of enacting." By theorizing on the "transgenerational mandate," Lebovici broached the question of the transmission of trauma and its impact in terms of risk for the development of the infant's "tree of life," his family tree, which has to house "ghosts" that do not belong to him. His therapeutic consultation model, following on the work by Winnicott [54], is a valuable framework in care strategies for mother–infant dyads in situations of severe distress.

In therapies for young children presenting disturbances linked to a psychologic trauma, transferential and countertransferential relationships frequently prove to be intense and violent. Transferential relations can be characterized by immediate and total attachment to the therapist, or, conversely, by complete opposition, whether passive or active. Countertransferential relations entail the risk of rejection, powerless rage, or, conversely, belief that the therapist is omnipotent. The different forms of countertransference are complex. They illustrate the empathy of the therapist and also point to that part of the trauma that is transferred. Indeed the authors hypothesize that what the therapist perceives in the countertransference is analogous to what is transferred to the infant. From work on traumatized mothers and infants, Lachal [55] has described emergent scenarios that he characterizes as a spontaneous response by the therapist to the narrative of the traumatic experience. For the therapist, this production of an "emergent scenario" is the sign of marked empathy at the time when the patient is absorbed in his or her narrative. The presence of this scenario is a sort of marker for a process of elaboration in the therapist, which likewise makes it possible for the patient. This is why the authors attach importance to the analysis of countertransference, both for mother–infant therapies and for individual and team group therapies.

Because these therapies are conducted in a transcultural situation, the authors pay particular attention to certain cultural factors: the language used, representations concerning the child and the disturbances the child presents, and possibilities for affiliation with a group or community [56].

To conclude, as suggested by Van Horn and Lieberman [57], the specific objectives of a parent–infant therapy in the context of trauma are

- Encouraging the abilities of the parents and the child to assess dangers and threats, to distinguish internal from external threats, and to respond in a suitable manner

- Developing the ability to regulate affects
- Restoring a feeling of confidence in bodily sensations and bodily exchanges between parents and child
- Restoring reciprocity: promoting intimate and affective exchanges between partners in the interaction
- Reassuring the child and parents as to the posttraumatic nature of experiences and feelings, by taking part in the early stages of the reconstruction of meaning
- Encouraging differentiation between traumatic reliving and remembering
- Placing the traumatic experience in its perspective as a part of the individual's experience and history, for which concern should diminish with time

A case study shows how the reinstatement of these processes gradually emerges in a transcultural situation.

A clinical history: Elavie

A Parisian maternity hospital made an emergency call to us concerning a situation about which they were worried and which clearly upset them. The care team was anxiously waiting for us and immediately presented a young woman who had arrived the previous night from Roissy airport, with no identification papers, confused, dazed, speaking very little French, and also pregnant. She was weeping and complaining of pains. She was urgently transported to the maternity hospital and gave birth 3 hours later.

I approached her bedside and found a slight young woman with very light skin, obviously scared, and completely immobile. I introduced myself and asked her if she spoke French. She seemed to understand but preferred to talk Lingala, her mother tongue. I was accompanied by an interpreter who is accustomed to working with me, and the rest of this first encounter was conducted in Lingala.

A war baby

The young mother is named Alfonsine and is barely 18. She weeps a lot during the interview, and more than anything she is afraid of being put onto a flight back to Congo. She says that if they send her back there she will be killed. She does not know exactly how she has got to where she is: a member of her family put her on a flight with a single ticket, without identification papers, and without telling her where she was going. I am struck by the fact that Alfonsine is not looking at her baby (a little girl) and asks no questions about her, even though she has just been born. She is clearly concerned about her own survival. I talk to her about the baby daughter—what name has she given? She tells me that the baby has no name as yet and adds: "This baby is a stranger." Alfonsine goes on, " If you want, you can give the baby a name, you can even give her your name; it will protect the baby." Alfonsine's interpretation of my concern for the baby girl as a mode of protection simultaneously shows her distress, her projected concern for the child, and her ability to lean on others for support, in particular on me. Where has this baby come from? Alfonsine replies that this is a "war baby," with no real father, and she bursts into tears hiding her face. The origin of the baby appears clear: the baby reminds her of a traumatic event, probably rape. All three adults fall silent, and the baby stops crying. On my instructions, the interpreter draws closer to her and suggests that the interview be terminated for today. Alfonsine then says that she wants the team to stay nearby but to stop talking. She then asks the team to carry the baby a little because her own arms are tired. The interpreter and I carry the baby around in turn—a small baby, very tonic and alert, who holds her head well and is seeking to suckle. The mother, who has dried her tears, watches the team members carrying the baby. For the first time there is a direct visual interaction between the mother and her baby. At this moment I recall Serge Lebovici often saying that the challenge is to convert the "capabilities" of the child into performance. Clearly this baby without a name is extremely capable, and shows it, but the mother cannot really see this. Perhaps she wants a nurse to give the baby some milk? She agrees: for the time being she wants the team to give this baby some milk in a bottle, "as they do in France," she remarks. In the last part of the encounter, when the baby is with the nurse, Alfonsine, terrified, tells the team of her fear of the night and darkness, that she is afraid of being touched, and that she has difficulty eating and often vomits. It all started about 9 months ago. She is from Brazzaville and fled the fighting with her mother and brothers. Her father stayed in Brazzaville. On the road one night they met some "militiamen" (the term she uses). The men raped her in front of her brothers and her mother, and then raped her mother. Her own rape was terrible, but it was even more terrible to see her mother raped; that is the experience that returns to her at night. The images of this event haunt her and return as soon as she closes her eyes. Her family continued on their way, even so. She was afraid she might have contracted AIDS, or that her mother had.

Life resumed; her body hurt, but life resumed—"it was possible" she says, astonished and frightened. It seems to me that in this "it was possible" there is a touch of wonder. Her mother told her that the main thing was to be together and alive. Then much later they all headed back toward Brazzaville. How much later? She does not remember. They all made their way back, except her mother, who died before, of old age, exhaustion, or something else. One night, when they were very close to Brazzaville, they met armed men along the road. One of them, she remembers, had a voice she knew, maybe a neighbor from home or someone she went to school with. She would rather not know. It was this man who raped her in front of her brothers. This time it was even harder. She screamed, asked them to kill her. After the rape she begged her brothers to leave her there and go on. She wanted to die; she wanted to be left alone. She wanted to rejoin her mother.

She has talked too much for today, she says. She does not want the team to go, she is afraid of being alone, she wants us to stay and remain silent. She looks at the interpreter and says: "You have a way of looking at me that is like my mother." This note that is at once poetic and transferential, moved me as much as my interpreter, taken aback by this sudden comparison. It moved me because it showed that this young mother had not lost her ability for dreaming. I begin to imagine her before the trauma: "Tell us about your mother." "My mother," she says, "married very young, a young man that she had chosen without her father's agreement. I was born from that."

The nurse brings the baby back, calm and satisfied, and she is put back in the cot near her mother. We suggest returning the next day to continue putting words to things. Clearly Alfonsine is suffering from a posttraumatic syndrome that expresses itself in her body, her sleep, her death wishes, her reminiscences. The repeated rapes, the rape of her mother, the loss of her mother, and perhaps other events, too, have left major sequelae. These sequelae affect her individual identity, her sexual identity, and her ability to become involved with a baby born from these circumstances.

Following this meeting, we initiate therapeutic consultations, long sessions of about 2 hours, but we do not always talk; sometimes, all four of us are quiet together. The baby punctuates the sessions. These consultations enable Alfonsine, first of all, to elaborate these extreme traumas that have left deep marks. Clearly some will affect her future destiny, but some can heal as long as they can find an acceptable inscription in her tree of life and will be transmissible without feelings of shame to her daughter.

For Alfonsine, the first stages are cathartic. She relates her traumatic memories with numerous details that sometimes are violent for the listener, too, because it is the mark of trauma to be traumatic to those hearing the narrative, of course to a lesser degree. The experience is not comparable, but the mark of the trauma exists for the other person in the encounter and even signals that an encounter has taken place. After the catharsis phase, the symptoms gradually alleviate but do not disappear completely. Then, in a second phase, she starts to ask what she is gong to do with the child: keep it, while it is the living incarnation of her rape? Give it up? Doing so, she says, will increase her shame even further.

This phase is followed by painstaking work on the tree of life of this baby. Alfonsine remembers her mother and summons her in her dreams. In the following interview she tells us that her mother "came to see her in the night" and that she wants her to keep the child with her.

A very "capable" baby

This baby looks well, I tell the baby so, as she looks at me, and I imagine she is smiling. (What does it matter if she is or not?) I observe furtive visual interaction between the mother and the baby and, above all, interactions involving touching and carrying: for the first time, Alfonsine has put the baby on her back, for a moment only; she did it because the baby was crying, and that soothed the child. I tell her what I see, and she smiles, hesitating to admit that she is breastfeeding. "Maybe that's why she looks so well," she says, almost jokingly. She began breastfeeding with a feeling of transgression mixed with guilt. She says later that she was afraid we would find her odd, breastfeeding a baby born from rape. This is the time when the relationship is forming, and early interactions are occurring that should not be missed because they contribute to the construction of parenthood.

Here we can see a basic mechanism at work in the early formation of the child's Self, which Lebovici propounded as early as 1961: the reciprocal investment between the child and the mother means that if the mother invests in her child, that investment has an effect on the mother which in turn alters the child's experience, and the same is true in reverse, for the child. This explains the primary importance of reciprocal investment and the fact that these constructions are necessary. There is an investment by the care team and by the authors' team in this little girl, and this investment draws out investment from the mother, leading her to reinvest in successive stages.

A little girl made human by milk and the ancestors

She is to give this little girl her mothers' name and her own milk. Her mother herself bore her maternal grandmother's name—a name that means "beginning." A little girl made human by milk and her ancestors, who will in return make her mother human, this mother who felt sullied by rape but consoled (her word) by the beauty of the child, by its capabilities, which she now perceives as performances, and by the child's very existence. She now will invest this child as a positive sign of destiny, after hesitating as to her meaning and the ties between them. She is asking more and more questions about the child's development. I ask a colleague psychologist to give her a development scale, the Brazelton scale for assessing abilities in infants. When the scale is administered, in my presence, it is a fine moment for Alfonsine, who is proud to see everything that this little girl is capable of. At times she has tears in her eyes. Later she tells me that the tears came when she thought of her mother. She is thinking that this little girl, born from horror, has come to console her after the death of her own mother. This is a first stage in the construction of the tree of life that gives the little girl a difficult, complex, ambivalent, but authentic place. From her existence, the roots can grow out. The child has played an active part, imposing herself by her vivacious energy and her ability to initiate interactions with her mother and the world.

In the interview that precedes her departure for a mother and infant home, Alfonsine tells me that she sometimes feels full of sad thoughts when she sees the baby, but that she feels she is a mother even so. And there is no doubt that this nascent maternal identity, hinged on the primary maternal concerns that are within her and filling her with a new feeling, will help her to restructure in another mode—deeply altered by the traumas but not annihilated, full of a painful otherness but able to invest in the future incarnated in this unwanted, unexpected, rejected baby that has come to be recognized as a part of herself and her history, however painful. She sometimes has feelings of anger when the baby cries at night, but she also remarks that they are the cries of life. The cries recall others, her own, but she now is able to differentiate meanings.

Alfonsine still lives in France. She has been able to find a cousin with whom she now lives with her daughter. Her daughter now has two first names: the first is "Lingala," and the second was added when she arrived at her cousin's. It was a name composed by all the women living around this child. The name they have given contains the notion of life and vitality (élan, vie)—"Elavie" [58].

Summary

Delivering appropriate care to refugee families requires complex care systems and models that take account of the social, cultural, and political dimensions as well as the psychologic (individual, interactional, family) dimension. In the social and political field, the impact of being recognized as a refugee is substantial. It can mean a new start with protected rights. The refusal of the designation "refugee" leads to the status of illegal migrant with the related risks and fears. In addition, the French integration model is based on individual rather than community integration, increasing the feeling of loneliness and abandonment. Sometimes, these patients can obtain an authorization to stay in the country for medical or psychologic reasons (with a medical certificate). In this context, they are not allowed to work. This situation creates a confusing contract between patient and doctor: as long as the patient is sick, he or she can obtain papers. The social work along side the psychologic work is essential and allows a therapeutic space to exist beyond the social concerns.

Support for parenting and parenthood and for the restoration of narrative and symbolization seem to the authors to be fundamental in the therapeutic process with parents and children. The babies born into these families, after events such as the families have experienced, are exposed to the consequences of their own past experiences and also, for those born after exile, to the transmission of the trauma experienced by their parents. This transmission of trauma can lead to alterations in these children's individual creative resources. This reality should lead therapists to ensure early care is provided for these families and their children, so that the transmission of the trauma and its consequences can be managed, avoiding serious damage. The goal is to provide care, in spite of all obstacles and difficulties.

References

[1] Rapport d'activité OFPRA. 2006. Available at: http://www.ofpra.gouv.fr/documents/rapport_Ofpra_2006.pdf. Accessed August 1, 2007.

[2] Moro MR, Lebovici S, editors. Psychiatrie humanitaire en ex-Yougoslavie et en Arménie. Paris: Presses Universitaires de France; 1995.

[3] Lachal C, Ouss-Ryngaert L, Moro MR, editors. Comprendre et soigner le trauma en situation humanitaire. Paris: Dunod; 2003.

[4] Moro MR. Parents en exil. Psychopathologie et migrations. Paris: PUF; 1994.

[5] Moro MR. Psychothérapie transculturelle des enfants de migrants. Paris: Dunod; 1998.

[6] Moro MR. Aimer ses enfants ici et ailleurs. Histoires transculturelles. Paris: Odile Jacob; 2007.

[7] Rezzoug D, De Plaën S, Bensekhar-Bennabi M, et al. Bilinguisme chez les enfants de migrants: mythes et réalités. Le Français Aujourd'hui 2007;158:61–8.

[8] Baubet T, Abbal T, Claudet J, et al. Traumas psychiques chez les demandeurs d'asile en France: des spécificités cliniques et thérapeutiques. Journal International de Victimologie 2004;2(2). [1 screen]. Available at: http://www.jidv.com/BAUBET,T-JIDV2004_%202(2).html. Accessed December 15, 2007.

[9] Fazel M, Stein A. The mental health of refugee children. Arch Dis Child 2002;87:366–70.

[10] Gonsalves CJ. Psychological stages of the refugee process: a model for therapeutic intervention. Prof Psychol Res Pr 1992;23:382–9.

[11] Lustig SL, Kia-Keating M, Knight WG, et al. Review of child and adolescent refugee mental health. J Am Acad Child Adolesc Psychiatry 2004;43(1):24–35.

[12] Papadopoulos RK. Refugees' families: issues of systemic supervision. Journal of Family Therapy 2001;23:207–13.

[13] Farwel N. Onward through strength: coping and psychological support among refugee youth returning to Eritrea from Sudan. J Refug Study 2001;14:1–69.

[14] Nathan T. La folie des autres. Traité d'ethnopsychiatrie clinique. Paris: Dunod; 1986.

[15] Nathan T. La fonction psychique du trauma. Nouvelle Revue d'ethnopsychiatrie 1987;7:7–10.

[16] American Psychological Association. Diagnostic and stastical manual of mental disorders. 3rd edition. Washington, DC: American Psychiatric Press; 1980.

[17] Lachal C, Moro MR. Treatment for sorrow. Medical News. 2002:11–16.

[18] Herman JL. Complex PTSD: a syndrome in survivors of prolonged and repeated trauma. J Trauma stress 1992;5(3):377–91.

[19] Van der Kolk BA. The complexity of adaptation to trauma. In: Van der Kolk BA, Mc Farlane AC, Weisaeth L, editors. Traumatic stress: the effect of overwhelming experiences on mind, body, and society. New York: Guilford Press; 1996. p. 182–213.

[20] Frey C. Post traumatic stress disorder and culture. In: Yilmaz AT, Weiss MG, Riecher-Rössler A, editors. Cultural psychiatry: euro-international perspectives. Basel (Switzerland): Karger; 2001. p. 103–16.

[21] Crocq L. Perspective historique sur le trauma. In: De Clerq M, Lebigot F, editors. Les traumatismes psychiques. Paris: Masson; 2001. p. 23–64.

[22] Taïeb O, Baubet T, Pradère J, et al. Traumatismes psychiques chez l'enfant et l'adolescent. EMC-Psychiatrie 2004;1(1):23–32.

[23] Freud A, Burlingham D. War and children. New York: International Universities Press; 1943.

[24] Freud A. Le traumatisme psychique. In: L'enfant dans la psychanalyse. Paris: Editions Gallimard; 1965. p. 205–14.

[25] Bailly L. Psychotraumatisme de l'enfant: avancées cliniques et théoriques. Nervure 1999;12: 20–5.

[26] Bailly L. Les guerres fratricides: quelles conséquences pour l'enfant? In: Maqueda F, editor. Les traumatismes de guerre. Revigny sur Ornain (France): Editions Hommes et Perspectives; 1999. p. 21–9.

[27] Bailly L. Traumatisme psychique chez le jeune enfant et théories sociales infantiles. In: Baubet T, Lachal C, Moro MR, editors. Bébés et trauma. France: La Pensée Sauvage Editions; 2003. p. 59–67.

[28] Winnicott DW. La crainte de l'effondrement. In: La crainte de l'effondrement et autres situations cliniques. Paris: Gallimard; 2000. p. 205–16.

[29] Winnicott DW. Le concept de traumatisme par rapport au développement de l'individu au sein de sa famille. In: La crainte de l'effondrement et autres situations cliniques. Paris: Gallimard; 2000. p. 292–312.

[30] Winnicott DW. Les enfants et la guerre. Paris: Payot; 2004.

[31] Scheeringa MS, Zeanah CH, Putman FW. New findings on alternative criteria for PTSD in preschool children. J Am Acad Child Adolesc Psychiatry 2003;42(5):561–70.

[32] Terr L. Childhood traumas: an outline and overview. Am J Psychiatry 1991;148(1):10–20.

[33] Bailly L. Les catastrophes et leurs conséquences psychotraumatiques chez l'enfant. Paris: Editions Soulas Francoises; 1996.

[34] Baubet T, Gaboulaud V, Grouiller K, et al. Facteurs psychiques dans les malnutritions infantiles en situation de post-conflit. Evaluation d'un programme de soins de dyades mères-bébés malnutris à Hébron (Territoires palestiniens). Ann Med Psychol (Paris) 2003;161:609–13.

[35] Lachal C. Le comportement de privation hostil. L'Autre Cliniques Cultures et Sociétés 2000; 1(1):77–89.

[36] Lachal C. La représentation de l'ennemi: penser l'autre pour se structurer. Champ Psychosomatique 1997;10:31–51.

[37] Mouchenik Y, Baubet T, Belanger F, et al. Evaluer les troubles psychologiques post-traumatiques chez les enfants de moins de six ans: à propos d'une étude réalisée à Debar (Macédoine). L'autre Cliniques Cultures Sociétés 2001;2(2):359–66.

[38] Drell MJ, Siegel CH, Gaensbauer TJ. Post traumatic stress disorder. In: Zeanah CH, editor. Handbook of infant mental health. New York: Guilford Press; 1993. p. 291–304.

[39] Scheeringa MS, Zeanah CH. A relational perspective on PTSD in early childhood. J Trauma Stress 2001;14:799–815.

[40] Lebigot F. L'effroi du traumatisme psychique:le regarder en face ou s'en protéger. Stress et Trauma 2002;2(3):139–46.

[41] Nathan T. Angoisse ou frayeur: un problème épistémologique de la psychanalyse. Nouv Rev Ethnopsychiatrie 1990;(15):21–38.

[42] Baubet T, Moro MR. Cultures et soins du trauma psychique en situation humanitaire. In: Baubet T, Le Roch K, Moro MR, editors. Soigner malgré tout. Trauma, cultures et soins, vol. 1. Grenoble (France): La Pensée Sauvage; 2003. p. 71–95.

[43] Rousseau C, Drapeau A. The impact of culture on the transmission of trauma. In: Danieli Y, editor. International handbook of multigenerational legacies of trauma. Norwell (MA): Kluwes International Publisher; 1998. p. 465–85.

[44] Zempléni A. La « maladie » et ses « causes ». Introduction [in French]. L'Ethnographie 1985; 81(2):13–44.

[45] Zempléni A. L'enfant Nit Ku Bon. Un tableau psychopathologique traditionnel chez les Wolof et les Lebou du Sénégal. Nouvelle Revue d'Ethnopsychiatrie 1985;4:9–42.

[46] Nathan T. L'enfant-ancêtre. Nouvelle Revue d'Ethnopsychiatrie 1985;4:7–9.

[47] Moro MR, Réal I. La consultation transculturelle d'Avicenne, Bobigny (France). In: Moro MR, De La Noë Q, Mouchenik Y, editors. Manuel de psychiatrie transculturelle: Travail clinique, travail social. Grenoble (France): La Pensée Sauvage; 2004. p. 217–38.

[48] Devereux G. (1972) Ethnopsychanalyse complémentariste. Paris: Flammarion; 1985.

[49] Baubet T, Marquer C, Sturm G, et al. Un dispositif original: le « groupe trauma ». Rhizome 2005;(21):33–7.

[50] Sturm G, Baubet T, Moro MR. Mobilizing social and symbolic resources in transcultural therapies with refugees and asylum seekers: the story of Mister Diallo. In: Drozdek B, Wilson P, editors. The voices of trauma: treating survivors across cultures. New York: Springer Science, Business Media, LLC; 2007. p. 211–32.

[51] Fonagy P, Steele H, Morans G, et al. Fantômes dans la chambre d'enfant: étude de la répercussion des représentations mentales des parents sur la sécurité de l'attachement. La Psychiatrie de l'Enfant 1996;39(1):63–83.

[52] Fonagy P. The transgenerational transmission of Holocaust trauma. Lessons learned from the analysis of an adolescent with obsessive-compulsive disorders. Attach Hum Dev 1999; 1(1):92–114.

[53] Lebovici S. Le nourrisson, sa mère et le psychanalyste. Les interactions précoces. Paris: Le Centurion; 1983.

[54] Winnicott DW. La consultation thérapeutique de l'enfant. Paris: Gallimard; 1971.

[55] Lachal C. Le partage du traumatisme. Contre-transferts avec les patients traumatisés. Grenoble (France): La Pensée Sauvage; 2006.

[56] Moro MR. Parents and infants in changing cultural context: immigration, trauma and risk. Infant Ment Health J 2003;24(3):240–64.

[57] Van Horn P, Lieberman AF. Early interventions with infants, toddlers, and preschoolers. In: Litz BT, editor. Early intervention for trauma and traumatic loss. New York: The Guilford Press; 2004. p. 112–30.

[58] Moro MR. Une clinique transculturelle. Elavie, un bébé de la guerre. PsychoMédia 2005;(7): 25–31.

ELSEVIER SAUNDERS

Child Adolesc Psychiatric Clin N Am
17 (2008) 569–584

CHILD AND
ADOLESCENT
PSYCHIATRIC CLINICS
OF NORTH AMERICA

Testimonials, Narratives, Stories, and Drawings: Child Refugees as Witnesses

Stuart L. Lustig, MD, MPH*,
Lakshika Tennakoon, MSc

*Department of Psychiatry, University of California San Francisco,
401 Parnassus Avenue, Box 0984F, San Francisco, CA, 94143, USA*

The United Nations Children's Fund (UNICEF) has estimated that 80% of war victims are women and children. In response to violence and political unrest, many people have been forced to flee their home countries in search of safety. There are in an estimated 19.2 million refugees and displaced people worldwide, approximately half of whom are children [1]. It is estimated that up to 40% of young refugees are vulnerable to developing mental health difficulties such as posttraumatic stress disorder (PTSD), depression, and other anxiety-related difficulties [2].

Although there are many treatments for traumatized refugee children, most notably cognitive behavior therapy and pharmacologic treatments that have been summarized elsewhere [3], the emerging literature on treatments involving narratives, testimonials, and story telling in this particular population has not been summarized. Studies on these types of treatments have emerged more slowly than the numerous studies quantifying the symptoms of PTSD and other psychiatric disorders that followed the inclusion of the PTSD diagnosis in the *Diagnostic and Statistical Manual of Mental Disorders*, third edition (DSM-III) in 1981. Indeed, although the impact of war trauma has long been recognized among combatants, the realization of the profound developmental impact of trauma on children is a relatively recent phenomenon, brought about in part by Terr's [4] longitudinal study involving the child survivors of the Chowchilla bus kidnapping in 1976. It is perhaps understandable that most studies of trauma among child refugees have focused on describing the phenomenology of psychiatric disorders or

* Corresponding author.
E-mail address: slustig@lppi.ucsf.edu (S.L. Lustig).

1056-4993/08/$ - see front matter. Published by Elsevier Inc.
doi:10.1016/j.chc.2008.02.001

childpsych.theclinics.com

on applying manualized treatments that target specific symptom profiles. As summarized by Miller and colleagues [5], however, narrative approaches to understanding trauma may offer the following advantages:

1. A deeper understanding of patterns of distress not captured by psychiatric nosology, such as cultural bereavement [6], and crises of meaning, identity, and faith [7], which are better understood by emic approaches that do not depend on medicalized disease constructs
2. A more comprehensive understanding of the timeline of events (as also described by Lustig and colleagues [8]) endured by refugees, a chronology insufficiently captured by static measurements of symptoms and social circumstances at just one or two time points
3. The opportunity to allow child refugees themselves to identify sources of stress and support, as opposed to an a priori assumption of factors that may or may not be applicable to the populations begin studied

In general, a narrative approach involves listening to the trauma story in a systematic way, and, in the case of testimonials, potentially using that story in a public venue for the purpose of education and advocacy. These stories also may be used in legal venues as legal testimony or in truth-and-reconciliation hearings. Testimonials were used first with survivors of Pinochet's regime in Chile in the 1970s [9] and again with Bosnian genocide survivors who were refugees in Chicago [10]. Meanwhile, narrative studies among adult patients who have PTSD have been summarized recently [11]. This article is limited largely to the use of narratives among those traumatized by war, particularly (but not exclusively) refugee children. Narrative studies of young refugees generally yield three kinds of information, depending on the study design. As will become apparent, some studies use narratives to generate content, which is analyzed by various qualitative means for the historical information contained within the narratives [12–14]. Another study focused on the syntax of the narrative as a function of trauma [15]. Although this study did not involve child refugees, these stories provide rich sources of data about the lives and experiences of child refugees. Still others evaluate the effectiveness of narratives in reducing symptoms or in attaining some other goal apart from generating historical content [16,17].

Methods

The state of the science in using narratives and testimonials was captured by two strategies: the psychiatric and psychologic literature was obtained from major databases such as PubMed, Medline, PsycINFO, and Web of Science using the key words "testimony," "narrative exposure," and "witnessing." The authors also performed a PubMed Mesh search using "narration" and "posttraumatic stress disorder." This search focused only on published literature in this field of research, rather than non–peer-reviewed or unpublished papers. Also, the references of recent review articles and white papers on the topic of child refugee mental health [18–20] were reviewed, and articles that seemed relevant were obtained. Any additional articles, projects, or initiatives of which the authors were aware were included also. The authors also searched the Web for summaries of art-based methods of story telling using the Google search engine and the search terms "drawings" and "refugee children."

Results

The authors identified 14 studies that addressed the use of testimonials or narrative therapy. These studies are summarized below and in Table 1. Because of the sparse published child-oriented research in this area, the authors have included studies of testimonial therapy among adult refugees or survivors of war.

As noted, studies of narratives and testimonials fall into three categories: (1) those whose primary purpose was to generate content about a specific type of experience (eg, flight from a war-torn area); (2) those that evaluated narratives or testimonials as a means of reducing symptoms; and (3) those that analyzed the structure of the narrative as a means of understanding the impact of the trauma.

Studies using narratives to generate content

The authors summarize two examples of testimonial psychotherapy with adults and then review reports of this method with children.

Van Dijk and colleagues [21] have used testimonial psychotherapy in the Netherlands with traumatized asylum seekers and refugees who have PTSD from Bosnia. The 12-session process, conducted by trained therapists with the help of interpreters where necessary, consisted of an introduction, psychoeducation, information on PTSD, an outline of the interviewee's life history, accounts of life before traumatic experiences took place, of traumatic experiences, life after traumatic experience, and current situations and expectations, reading and editing the document, signing the document, and termination.

Agger and Jensen [22] presented verbatim transcriptions of several sessions of testimony provided by a 25-year-old African male refugee and a 30-year-old Middle Eastern male refugee, both residing in Denmark. Although the methodology for testimony as described among adults, such as the means of eliciting the narrative and the number of sessions, may need to be adapted for child refugee populations, the conceptual basis is adaptable. Conceptually, the authors noted that testimony may work best among refugees who have an ideological commitment to documenting wrongdoing. Such a process may have psychologic benefits such as alleviating survivor guilt [23].

Table 1
Summary of studies of narratives, testimony, and storytelling

Author [reference]	Country of origin	Study population	Study design	Sample Size	Assessments and treatments	Outcomes
Van Dijk, et al [21]	The Netherlands	Patients are asylum seekers or legal refugees in the Netherlands and war victims	Conceptual review on testimony therapy	—	Testimony therapy	Feasible and effective method at reducing symptoms
Berman, et al [14]	Canada	Refugee women exposed to war	Narrative research design	9	Review of narratives	Experiences of pain and suffering were shared equally regardless of the trauma.
Agger and Jensen [22]	Denmark	African and Middle Eastern male asylum cases	Case histories	2	Testimony method	Testimony method may help reduce the symptoms.
Goodman [12]	United States	Sudanese male refuges in United States	Case-centered; comparative narrative approach	14	Narratives	Identified four themes used as coping strategies: (1) collectivity and the communal self, (2) suppression and distraction, (3) making meaning, (4) emerging from hopelessness to hope.
Lustig, et al [13]	United States	Sudanese refugees in Boston	Case series	3	Testimonial psychotherapy	Testimonial psychotherapy is safe, acceptable, and feasible in adolescent refugees.
Neuner, et al [28]	Germany	Kosovan refugee in a Macedonian refugee camp	Case-report	1	NET, PDS	Reduction of PTSD symptoms occurred after three NET sessions.

Study	Country	Population	Study type	n	Measures	Findings
Neuner, et al [16]	Germany	Sudanese refugees who had PTSD	Randomized, controlled study of NET, SC, and PE	43	DFMQ, SRQ-20, PDS	Greater reduction of PTSD symptoms seen after NET than after SC or PE.
Onyut, et al [17]	Germany	Somali children living in a refugee settlement in Uganda	Case reports; pilot study	6	CIDI, NET at baseline and follow-up at 9 months	Posttreatment symptom reduction at baseline and 9-month follow-up
Igreja, et al [33]	Mozambique	Mozambican civil war survivors	Randomized study	206	SRQ, HTQ, NITE, SIFP Testimony intervention	Symptom reduction reported in the intervention and control group.
Onyut, et al [37]	Germany	Rwandan, Somalian, Burundian, Sudanese, and Ethiopian refugees in Uganda refugee camp	Intervention study of NET or supportive counseling Epidemiologic survey.	1473	PDS, DSM-IV, CIDI, HSCL-25	Prevalence of chronic PTSD ranging from 31.1% to 47%.
Schauer, et al [30]	Germany	Based on severely traumatized 13-year-old Somali refugee	Case history	1	NET	PTSD symptoms were reduced; reduction in avoidance, and intrusive symptoms
O'Kearney and Perrott [11]	Australia	Review of nature of trauma narratives in PTSD	Review article	6	–	Evidence for PTSD-related narrative fragmentation was inconclusive.
Kenardy, et al [15]	Australia	Children who had experienced a physical injury trauma	Follow-up study 6 months from baseline	87	ADIS-P, DSM-IV child version	Weak association between dissociative trauma narrative themes and PTSD
Hanney and Kozlowska [39]	Australia	Based on healing traumatized children	Review	–	–	Development of trauma-specific interventions associated with drawings and illustrated stories

Abbreviations: ADIS-P, Anxiety Disorders Interview Schedule-Parent interview; CIDI, Composite International Diagnostic Interview; DFMQ, Demography of Forced Migration Questionnaire; DSM-IV, Diagnostic and Statistical Manual of mental Disorders, fourth edition; HSCL-25, Hopkins Symptom Checklist; HTQ, Harvard Trauma Questionnaire; NET, narrative exposure therapy; NITE, Nocturnal Intrusions after Traumatic Experiences Questionnaire; PDS, Posttraumatic Stress Diagnostic Scale; PE, psychoeducation; PTSD, posttraumatic stress disorder; SC, supportive counseling; SRQ, self-reporting questionnaire.

Goodman [12] conducted a case series among 14 male Sudanese adolescent refugees residing in the Boston area. The author interviewed and audiotaped them in English with an unstructured interview guide consisting of broad, open-ended questions designed to elicit participants' stories. Transcriptions were analyzed for content, theme, and structure. Participants' narratives were replete with the horrors and suffering (eg, violence, death, hunger, and thirst) during the long civil war between the northern and southern parts of Sudan. In addition to the danger and constant hardship, they also talked about different coping strategies they used to survive. Four emerging themes highlighted these strategies: (1) collectivity and the communal self, (2) suppression and distraction, (3) making meaning, and (4) emerging from hopelessness to hope. Most of the study participants reported feeling safe for the first time since they had left their families in Africa. A potential limitation of the study was that narratives from these Sudanese boys were elicited by a middle-aged, white woman in the United States, and results may have differed had participants been telling their stories to someone of their age, gender, or cultural group.

Lustig and colleagues [13] performed a case series study among a smaller subset of this Sudanese adolescent cohort in Boston. Following an initial focus group with the sponsoring foster agency (Lutheran Social Services) and key members of the Sudanese and parent community involved in the boys' lives, the authors approached eight Sudanese adolescent refugees and recruited the first three boys who volunteered to take part of the study. The participants first completed a guided relaxation exercise and then were interviewed and audiotaped in English over the course of three to nine 1-hour sessions, the number of sessions being determined by the subjects. Final testimonies ranged from 11 to 33 pages, which the subjects were actively engaged in editing. Narrative themes included the importance of family, religious conviction, and education. A subsequent focus group with subjects found testimonial psychotherapy to be an acceptable, safe, and feasible therapeutic approach for an adolescent refugee population. Participants emphasized that the desire to share their stories to improve life back in Sudan was a strong motivation for their involvement.

Berman and colleagues [14] performed a narrative study of refugee women who had experienced violence in the context of war. The study sample, located in Canada, consisted of nine women, including three from Bosnia, three from Guatemala, two from El Salvador, and one from Chile. A semistructured interview guide was used that consisted of open-ended questions about aspects of women's lives before, during, and after migration to Canada. Interviews were conducted in either English or Spanish. Analysis, according to the methods of Mishler [24] and Riessman [25], entailed retranscribing sections of text that seemed to take a narrative form and reducing them to the core narrative for coding and sorting. Participants reported both direct and indirect exposure to violence. Eight themes that emerged were lives forever changed; new notions of normality; a pervasive sense of fear; selves obscured; living among and between cultures; a women's place in Canada; bearing heavy burdens and the centrality of children; and perceptions of an uncaring system of care.

Studies of symptom reduction or functional improvement

Based on the principles of testimonial psychotherapy, narrative exposure therapy (NET) has been developed and propagated by the Vivo ("*Vic*tim's *Vo*ice") Foundation [26]. Narrative therapy involves the iterative construction of an autobiographic memory and a consistent narrative which, it is hypothesized, fosters habituation to emotional responses (with reduced symptoms upon recall) and prevents fragmentation of traumatic memories. Participants often are pleased to have their narratives contribute to the collective documentation process of human rights abuses (eg, posting the stories on a human rights organization Website) [27].

As in the previous section, the authors here summarize two adult studies (case reports using NET with adults, followed by a larger adult study of NET) and then discuss a version adapted for child refugees. Neuner and colleagues [28] used NET to treat a 24-year-old woman in a Macedonian refugee camp during the Balkan war. Her dissociative symptoms were identified by the Posttraumatic Stress Diagnostic Scale (PDS) [29]. After three sessions, each lasting about 70 minutes, her mood was improved dramatically. Re-experiencing symptoms decreased from a score of 15 to 5, arousal decreased from a score of 15 to 9, and avoidance decreased from a score of 18 to 8.

As is typical of the downward extension to child populations of psychiatric treatments that are promising in adults, Schauer and colleagues [30] discussed a case study based on NET with a child, subsequently called "KIDNET." The authors developed KIDNET as a child-friendly exposure treatment. Because children are not as capable as adults of articulating their stories verbally, the authors used theater and illustrative materials (eg, the "life-line exercise") during NET treatment sessions. Specifically, a rope represented the child's lifeline. Flowers were placed alongside the rope to mark the positive life experiences, and stones were used to mark the negative ones. These materials helped the child to reconstruct memories of his or her experiences. The case study described a 13-year-old Somalian boy living in a refugee camp in Uganda, who had PTSD and who received four sessions of KIDNET, each ranging from 60 to 90 minutes, over a 3-week period. The posttreatment findings revealed that the participant had not been exposed to additional traumatic events (an important consideration for refugees still living in a perilous environment), and the score for PTSD symptoms on the PDS dropped from 36 (the maximum possible score is 51) before the intervention to 12 over a 6-month period.

Neuner and colleagues [16] performed a comparison study of NET, supportive counseling, and psychoeducation for the treatment of PTSD among Sudanese refugees living in a refugee settlement in Uganda. The authors selected 77 participants from a list of respondents who previously had been selected randomly for a survey. Forty-three (56%) had diagnoses of PTSD according to DSM IV criteria [31] as diagnosed by expert interviewers using the Composite International Diagnostic Interview (CIDI) [32] and were included in the study. Subjects were assigned randomly to one of three different treatment approaches: NET (n = 17), supportive counseling (n = 14), or psychoeducation (n = 12). The participants received treatment for a year. Only 29% of the NET group but 79% of supportive counseling group and 80% of the psychoeducation group fulfilled the PTSD criteria after 1 year of treatment. It bears explicit mention that this study, in contrast to others presented earlier, was conducted in a refugee settlement community on the African continent rather than in a postmigration country. The authors noted that participants' receipt of the written biography upon completion, even if they could not understand the English text, was a unique motivator, as was the desire to have testimonies published to educate the world about the Sudanese civil war.

Igreja and colleagues [33] evaluated the effectiveness and feasibility of testimony to reduce PTSD symptoms among 206 participants living in an agricultural community in Mozambique, all of whom had been affected by the war in their country. The study population divided into two groups including a case (n = 137) and a noncase group (n = 69) based on the data collected with the Self-Report Questionnaire (SRQ) [34] for psychiatric morbidity, the Harvard Trauma Questionnaire [35] for traumatic experiences, the Nocturnal Intrusions after Traumatic Experiences questionnaire [36] for the presence of nightmares, and the Self-Inventory for PTSD, for PTSD symptoms. The case group (n = 137) was assigned randomly to an intervention group (n = 66) or a control group (n = 71). The intervention and control groups did not differ in demographic variables or in exposure to trauma. The authors assessed symptoms at baseline, after intervention, and at a follow-up 11 months later. The intervention group received testimony intervention in the native Chi-Gorongose language with native-language interpreters who were the same gender as the participants. The testimonies were structured to include the following elements: details about a major traumatic experience and the person's role and perceptions at the time, including the social dimensions of the experience; perceptions and feelings at the time of the testimony; the relationship between the experience and the present situation; and feelings about the future. The testimonies were written in note form, and the interviewer read the testimony back to the participants to obtain an accurate final version. The control group did not receive any intervention. For all measurements, in both the intervention and control groups, each individual's postintervention score was significantly than the baseline score, but no greater symptom reduction was noted in the intervention group. Combining both groups at the 11-month follow-up point, SRQ scales had dropped significantly, as had scores on the hyperarousal subscale of the Self-Inventory for PTSD. In explaining the absence of a specific treatment effect over time between the intervention and control group, the authors noted that for most participants, testimony was given in only one session, and that a great deal of interaction and communication among all community members may have diluted any effect of this session among the intervention group.

Onyut and colleagues [37] investigated the utility of short-term treatment strategies, NET, and supportive counseling in a disaster region by recruiting and training local paramedical personnel. Adults and children were screened with the PDS for PTSD diagnoses, which was validated with the CIDI (World Health Organization, 1997) [32]. The Hopkins Symptom Checklist-25 (HSC-25) [38] was used to screen for depression. More than 100 subjects who had PTSD were included in the study. Both NET and supportive counseling were conducted for four to six sessions by a same-sex therapist for each client. Each session lasted 1 to 2 hours. At the end of therapy patients assigned to NET therapy and supportive counseling received either a documented account of their lives or a case summary, respectively.

The authors are not aware of a report for the adults in the study, but results were reported separately for six Somali children suffering from PTSD [17]. At baseline, the children met criteria for PTSD, and four met criteria for depression. Participants received four to six individual sessions of KIDNET. Symptoms were reduced immediately after the KIDNET treatment and at follow-up. Although only four subjects were available for testing immediately following the intervention, all were available for follow-up at 9 months. The follow-up interviews were conducted using the PDS and the HSC-25 and were validated with the CIDI. Initial moderate to severe trauma scores (mean = 14.3; SD = 1.9) dropped to 9.0 (SD = 2.2) at posttest and again to 6.2 (SD = 3.3) at 9 months' follow-up. By 9 months, four of the six patients no longer met criteria for PTSD, and the other two had borderline scores. Of the four patients who initially met criteria for depression at baseline, none met these criteria at 9 months. The authors concluded that KIDNET is a safe, feasible treatment for PTSD in children. This study had no control group, but the authors proposed that spontaneous remission of symptoms was unlikely, given the high prevalence of PTSD in the Somali refugee population.

Studies focused on narrative syntax as a function of trauma

The authors identified only one study of narrative structure and syntax in children (but none among refugees), which they present here following a synopsis of a recently published review of such studies among traumatized adults. Although not focused on child refugees, these studies illustrate the type of research that theoretically is feasible with child refugees. Specifically, O'Kearney and Perrott [11] reviewed 19 studies of trauma narratives to examine a relationship between trauma narratives and psychopathology and adjustment. They included relevant articles identified in MEDLINE,

PsycINFO, and EMBASE using the search key words "trauma narratives," "trauma memory," "narrative and PTSD," "language and PTSD," and "narrative and therapy."

Thirteen of the 19 studies assessed linguistic indices coded from the trauma narratives, six studies used participants' ratings of narrative or memory quality, and three studies used both types of measures. Traumas experienced were heterogeneous across the studies. The time frame since the time of trauma ranged from a few days to years. The reviewers focused on the following narrative components: sensory, perceptual, or emotional dominance; narrative disorganization or fragmentation; disruptive temporal context; and the nature of references to self. Findings showed a relative dominance of sensory/perceptual emotional language in PTSD trauma narratives and a relationship between this type of language and peritraumatic dissociation and the "flashback" quality of the memories. The relationship between self-referential themes or narrative disorganization was found to be less predictive of PTSD, however. The evidence for PTSD-related narrative fragmentation was inconclusive. The study authors pointed out that the poor validity and the confusion of content and syntactic aspects of narrative organization limited the data on PTSD narratives.

The relationship between children's trauma narrative themes and future trauma symptoms was investigated by Kenardy and colleagues [15]. Participants were 87 children aged 7 to 15 years who had experienced a physical injury trauma and who were recruited from the accident and emergency centers at three hospitals in southeast Queensland in Australia. The authors assessed the study population with the Anxiety Disorders Interview Schedule for DSM-IV–Child Version, Parent Interview Schedule to measure anxiety, PTSD, and other emotional and behavioral disorders. Interviewers conducted a home visit 4 to 7 weeks after the trauma, during which verbal narratives of the child's injury were recorded on audiotape. Among participants, 35.6% of the narratives were coded as having absence of emotion, and 47.1% of children were identified as presenting dissociation in their narrative by the presence of temporal disorganization or dissociative amnesia or the absence of emotion. Children who reported longer narratives were more likely to show temporal disorganization. Children who showed temporal disorganization in narrative themes, but not absence of emotion or dissociative amnesia, were more likely to report concurrent subsyndromal PTSD symptoms. Only weak associations were noted between dissociative trauma narrative themes and PTSD.

The use of storybooks and drawings

In a conceptual paper based, in part, on two case vignettes, Hanney and Kozlowska [39] conducted a review on healing methods for traumatized children. They noted that illustrated stories offer a predictable structure to sessions and facilitate the engagement and participation of children in therapy. The authors discussed the therapeutic properties of storybooks, namely that they can take into account a specific child's life story, verbal capacity, level of anxiety, and traumatic hyperarousal. The authors noted that artwork can help create coherent narratives and family stories about a traumatic past and that creating art is a generally pleasant process that provides an experience contrary to that associated with trauma and therefore facilitates desensitization and processing of traumatic memories. They developed the "illustrated storybook" for children age 3 through 14 years on an inpatient child psychiatry unit who presented with complex histories of trauma [40]. A visual autobiographic strategy such as this provides youngsters the opportunity to rework views about themselves in a way that does not depend on language and that may foster the expression of nondeclarative memories among very young children.

Drawings by refugee children, as a window into their world, are available on the Web. For example, CareBridge is a cooperative of relief, sustainability, and information technology organizations dedicated to whole-systems, community-based design and development for displaced populations. In the Foreign and Commonwealth Office Visitors' Center it showcases a selection of drawings by Kosovar Albanian children ages 6 through 9 years from a Macedonia refugee camp. Examples of refugee children's drawings are viewable at http://www.globalsecurity.org/military/ops/kosovo-990505-drawings.htm. They depict scenes of tanks and guns, policemen with knives, houses on fire, and dead people lying in the road with blood next to them. The children were not asked to draw these pictures; rather, they used the opportunity of an art class to express what they had seen and survived.

Meanwhile, on mission along the border of Chad and Darfur, Human Rights Watch researchers gave children notebooks and crayons to keep them occupied while they spoke with the children's parents. Without any instruction or guidance, the children drew scenes from their experiences of the war in Darfur: the attacks by the Janjaweed, the bombings by Sudanese government forces, the shootings, the burning of entire villages, and the flight to Chad. These drawings are available at http://hrw.org/photos/2005/darfur/drawings/index.htm.

The Children Left Behind project is a collaboration of Catholic Relief Services and Capitol Children's Museum. Catholic Relief Services is the official international relief and development agency of the Catholic community in the United States. The drawings are based on Afghan refugee children who reside in Shamshatoo refugee camp in Pakistan. Their drawings are available at http://www.thechildrenleftbehind.org/previous.htm. They suggest that children desire to represent and understand the experiences they have gone through, using the representational tools at their disposal.

Discussion

Mental health professionals play a critical role in the early detection of problems and the treatment of child and adolescent refugees. It is important to identify cases as early as possible to plan an appropriate intervention to reduce the burdensome symptoms, which might affect the child's adjustment, schooling, and home life.

The desire to hear stories and to tell them is universal. Young children working through the typical struggles of child development use stories to work and rework intrapsychic conflicts on a regular basis, often asking for the same bedtime story again and again [41]. The authors found several studies that capitalized on this innate interest in narratives to provide order and meaning for events that were far more catastrophic than those of a typical childhood.

Of note, many studies involve someone who may be identified as "different" from those telling their stories: different ethnicities, races, genders, nationalities. The impact of these differences on the storytelling process is unknown, as is any affect on the content, the healing process, and the person's own role in the story. Another common theme was the eventual use of the testimonies that were of significant interest to those testifying. An unanswered question is how much therapeutic benefit is attributable to telling the story initially versus organizing it versus having someone listen to and disseminate it.

From the literature, which is sparse thus far, one can conclude that the narrative methods reviewed here, namely testimonial psychotherapy, NET, storybooks, and drawings, are at least feasible. Symptom reduction was noted in a handful of studies, although testimony was not superior to no treatment in one [33] of two randomized studies. It would seem that the field is ripe for more comprehensive efficacy studies of testimonials, narratives, and storytelling in both war-torn areas and countries of resettlement.

The unique qualities of testimonials that yield a written document to educate the world, a strong motivation for participants in several studies, reduce the problems of treatment fidelity that plague psychotherapy studies in general. The use of testimonial therapy begs the question about the obligations of the listener actually to use the testimony for its intended purpose. Additionally, researchers probably will need to include an informed consent process for the intended uses of the testimonials obtained from participants.

Timing and location are important considerations. All three testimonial studies that focused on the generation of content found that participants acknowledged significant suffering and were able to think deeply about their experiences. Less is known, however, about the extent to which these abilities depend on the safety of the setting. For example, would settings other than postmigration settings work as well? Only a few of the studies included in this review were conducted in refugee camps [16,17,28,37]. Also, is there an optimal time period after index traumas during which to take testimony?

Although there are aspects of all narrative therapies that could be therapeutic, the particular meaning-making device of producing a story to transform private pain into spiritual dignity [22] makes testimonies and narratives unique and therefore perhaps easier to quantify as more or less effective than other, less distinguishable types of therapy.

Interest in the stories of children extends far beyond the confines of academic child psychiatry and psychology. *Anne Frank: The Diary of a Young Girl* has been required reading for generations of school children. The lay public has eagerly purchased copies of Dave Eggers' *What is the What, The Autobiography of Valentino Achak Deng: A Novel* [42]. This "shattering work of testimony" [43] is a fictionalized account of one young Sudanese man's heroic trek through the treacherous deserts of Sudan, Ethiopia, and Kenya, much of it narrated from the floor of his gritty inner-city Atlanta apartment where his muggers have tied him down for several hours of retraumatizing captivity. Although the novel is filled with accurate historical details, the "liberties and devices of fiction," such as dialogue, voice, and characterization, enable a remarkably vivid rendering of a complex story of human suffering [44]. Another narrative from Africa, *A Long Way Gone from Home: Memoirs of a Child Soldier*, by Beah [45], traces the author's journey from Sierra Leone, where he was a child soldier, to New York where he was adopted by a white Jewish American woman, to Oberlin College. Although *Time* commented on the "cultural sweet spot for the African child soldier," and *Mother Jones* noted "that this is the year child soldiers went pop"[46], readers have been educated and moved by the these young authors.

Refugee children also are among the intended beneficiaries of the Our Stories project, an initiative that Google, in partnership with the One Laptop Per Child (OLPC) Foundation [47] (as well as with UNICEF and others), hopes to roll out by the time this article is published. The collaboration is placing audiorecording capabilities and interviewing lessons on laptops provided to school children in developing countries, to allow them to generate stories from their friends, families, and others in their community as a way of sharing their lives with the world. Through OLPC, school children in developing countries are receiving durable, easy-to-use laptop computers that will be networked with fellow students and other OLPC schools, so that "all school-aged children in the developing world are able to engage effectively with their own personal laptop, networked to the world, so that they, their families and their communities can openly learn and learn about learning" (Laura Bergheim of Google, personal communication, 2007).

Summary

Based on the state of the science of testimonial narrative, storytelling, and drawings among refugees, the authors offer the following recommendations:

1. For testimonial and narrative techniques, move beyond feasibility studies to evaluate efficacy in randomized, controlled trials.
2. Ensure that studies in war-torn areas provide a research setting that is as safe as possible for participants and that they do not fear retribution of any type as a result of the stories they share.

3. For regions in which the Internet is a preferred means communicating, consider using Websites as a way to share completed stories and ensure linkages with other Websites to ensure maximum visibility.
4. For young children, use nonverbal methods, including artwork and physical objects, to facilitate talking about one's life; these techniques also need further study of their efficacy, particularly among refugee children.

Reference

[1] United Nations High Commission for Refugees. 2004 Global refugee trends. Overview of refugee populations, new arrivals, durable solutions, stateless and other persons of concern to UNHCR. Geneva (Switzerland): United Nations High Commission for Refugees; 2005.

[2] Hodes M. Psychologically distressed refuge children in the United Kingdom. Child Psychology and Psychiatry Review 2000;5:57–68.

[3] Ehntholt K, Yule W. Practitioner review: assessment and treatment of refugee children and adolescents who have experienced war related trauma. J Child Psychol Psychiatry 2006;12: 1197–210.

[4] Terr LC. Too scared to cry how trauma affects children and ultimately us all. New York: Basic Books; 1976.

[5] Miller KE, Worthington GJ, Muzurovic J, et al. Bosnian refugees and the stressors of exile: a narrative study. Am J Orthopsychiatry 2002;72(3):341–54.

[6] Eisenbruch M. Can homesickness kill? In: Abbott M, editor. Refugee settlement and well-being. Auckland (New Zealand): Mental Health Foundation of New Zealand; 1988. p. 101–17.

[7] Silove D. The psychosocial effects of torture, mass human rights violations, and refugee trauma. J Nerv Ment Dis 1999;187(4):200–7.

[8] Lustig S, Kia-Keating M, Knight WG, et al. Review of child and adolescent refugee mental health. J Am Acad Child Adolesc Psychiatry 2003;443(1):24–36.

[9] Cienfuegos AJ, Monelli C. The testimony of political repression as a therapeutic instrument. Am J Orthopsychiatry 1983;53:43–51.

[10] Weine SM, Dzubur Kelanvic A, Pavkovic I, et al. Testimony psychotherapy with Bosnian refugees: a pilot study. Am J Psychiatry 1998;155(12):1720–6.

[11] O'Kearney J, Perrott K. Trauma narratives in posttraumatic stress disorder: a review. J Trauma Stress 2006;19(1):91–3.

[12] Goodman J. Coping with trauma and hardship among unaccompanied refugee youths from Sudan. Qual Health Res 2004;14(9):1177–96.

[13] Lustig S, Weine S, Saxe G, et al. Testimonial psychotherapy for adolescent refugees: a case series. Transcult Psychiatry 2004;41(1):31–45.

[14] Berman H, Girón ER, Marroquín AP. A narrative study of refugee women who have experienced violence in the context of war. Can J Nurs Res 2006;38(4):32–53.

[15] Kenardy J, Smith A, Spence SH, et al. Dissociation in children's trauma narratives: an exploratory investigation. J Anxiety Disord 2007;21:456–66.

[16] Neuner F, Schauer M, Klaschik C, et al. A comparison of narrative exposure therapy, supportive counseling and psychoeducation for treating posttraumatic stress disorder in an African refugee settlement. J Consult Clin Psychol 2004;72(No 4):579–87.

[17] Onyut LP, Neuner F, Schauer E, et al. Narrative exposure therapy as a treatment for child was survivors with posttraumatic stress disorder: two case reports and a pilot study in an African refugee settlement. BMC Psychiatry 2005;5(7):1–9.

[18] Barenbaum J, Ruchkin V, Schwab-Stone M. The psychosocial aspects of children exposed to war: practice and policy initiatives. J Child Psychol Psychiatry 2004;45(1):41–62.

[19] The National Child Traumatic Stress Network. Mental health interventions for refugee children in resettlement. White paper II from the National Child Traumatic Stress Network Refugee Trauma Task Force. Available at: www.NCTSNet.org. Accessed March 18, 2008.

[20] The National Child Traumatic Stress Network. Review of child and adolescent refugee mental health. White paper from the National Child Traumatic Stress Network Refugee Trauma Task Force. Available at: www.NCTSN.org. Accessed March 18, 2008.

[21] Van Dijk J, Schoutrop M, Spinhoven P. Testimony therapy: treatment method for traumatized victims or organized violence. Am J Psychother 2003;57:361–73.

[22] Agger I, Jensen B. Testimony as a ritual and evidence in psychotherapy for political refugees. J Trauma Stress 1990;3(No 1):115–30.

[23] Danieli T. Treating survivors and children of survivors of the Nazi holocaust. In: Ochberg FM, editor. Post traumatic therapy and victims of violence. New York: Brunner/Mazel; 1988. p. 278–94.

[24] Mishler E. The analysis of interview-narratives. In: Sarbin TR, editor. Narrative psychology 1986. The storied nature of human conduct. New York: Praeger; 1986. p. 233–55.

[25] Riessman CK. Narratives analysis. Newbury Park (CA): Sage; 1993.

[26] Available at: www.vivofoundation.net. Accessed March 18, 2008.

[27] Braiker B, Rocklin P, Ayotte B, et al. Stories of survival: Asylum seekers in Amercia: testimonial therapy: Three stories from Sudan. Available at: http://physiciansforhumanrights.org/asylum/stories/testimonial-therapy/. Accessed March 18, 2008.

[28] Neuner F, Schauer M, Roth W, et al. A narrative exposure treatment as intervention in a refugee camp: a case report. Behavioral and Cognitive Psychotherapy 2002;30:205–9.

[29] Foa EB. Post-traumatic Stress Diagnostic Scale (PDS). Minneapolis (MN): National Computer Systems; 1995.

[30] Schauer E, Neuner F, Elbert T, et al. Narrative exposure therapy in children: a case study. Intervention 2004;1(2):18–32.

[31] American Psychiatric Association. Diagnostic and statistical manual of mental disorders. 4th edition. Washington, DC: American Psychiatric Association; 1994.

[32] World Health Organization. Composite International Diagnostic Interview (CIDI). Geneva (Switzerland): World Health Organization; 1997.

[33] Igreja V, Kleijn WC, Schreuder BJN, et al. Testimony method to ameliorate post-traumatic stress symptoms. Community based intervention study with Mozambican civil war survivors. Br J Psychiatry 2004;184:251–7.

[34] Harding T, de Arango M, Baltazar J, et al. Mental disorders in primary health care: a study of their frequency and diagnosis in developing countries. Psychol Med 1980;10:231–41.

[35] Mollica R, Caspi Yavin Y, Lavelle J, et al. Harvard Trauma Questionnaire (HTQ): manual of Cambodian, Laotian and Vietnamese versions. Torture Quarterly: Journal on Rehabilitation of Torture Victims and Prevention of Torture 1996;(Suppl 1):19–42.

[36] Schreuder B, Kleijn W, Rooijmans H. Nocturnal re-experiencing more than forty years after war trauma. J Trauma Stress 2000;23:453–63.

[37] Onyut L, Neuner F, Schauer E, et al. The Nakivale Camp Mental Health Project: building local competency for psychological assistance to traumatized refugees. Intervention 2004;2: 90–107.

[38] Derogaits LR, Lipman RS, Rickels K, et al. COVI: the Hopkins Symptom Checklist (HSCL): a self report symptom inventory. Behav Sci 1974;1–15.

[39] Hanney L, Kozlowska K. Healing traumatized children: creating illustrated storybooks in family therapy. Fam Process 2002;41:37–65.

[40] Kozlowska K, Hanney L. An art therapy group for children traumatized by parental violence and separation. Clin Child Psychol Psychiatry 2001;6:49–78.

[41] Bettelheim B. The ues of enchantment. The meaning and importance of fairy tales. New York: Vintage Books; 1977.

[42] Eggers D. What is the what. The autobiography of Valentino Achak Deng. A novel. San Francisco (CA): McSweeney's; 2006.

[43] Freeman J. Eggers shadows a boy out of Africa. A tragicomic tale that revolves around a riddle. Boston Globe Dec 17, 2006. Available at: http://www.boston.com/ae/books/articles/2006/12/17/eggers_shadows_a_boy_out_of_. Accessed March 18, 2008.

[44] Prose P. The lost boy. New York Times Book Review September 24, 2006. p. 1, 6.

[45] Beah I. A long way gone from home: memoirs of a child soldier. Sarah Crichton Books; 2007.

[46] Court A. The child soldiers of Staten Island. Mother Jones June 30th, 2007. Available at: http://www.motherjones.com/commentary/columns/2007/07/witness.html. Accessed March 18, 2008.

[47] One laptop per child: Mission. Available at: www.laptop.org. Accessed March 18, 2008.

ELSEVIER
SAUNDERS

Child Adolesc Psychiatric Clin N Am
17 (2008) 585–604

CHILD AND
ADOLESCENT
PSYCHIATRIC CLINICS
OF NORTH AMERICA

Cognitive Behavioral Therapy for Symptoms of Trauma and Traumatic Grief in Refugee Youth

Laura K. Murray, PhD[a],*, Judith A. Cohen, MD[b],
B. Heidi Ellis, PhD[c], Anthony Mannarino, PhD[d]

[a]*Boston University School of Public Health, Center for International Health and Development, 85 E. Concord Street, 5th Floor, Boston, MA 02118, USA*
[b]*Center for Traumatic Stress in Children & Adolescents, Department of Psychiatry, Allegheny General Hospital and Drexel University College of Medicine, 4 Allegheny Center, 8th Floor, Pittsburgh, PA 15212, USA*
[c]*Children's Hospital Center for Refugee Trauma, Children's Hospital Boston, 300 Longwood Avenue, Boston, MA 02115, USA*
[d]*Department of Psychiatry, Allegheny General Hospital, Drexel University College of Medicine, Four Allegheny Center, Pittsburgh, PA 15212, USA*

Over time, wars and disasters have increasingly targeted or involved civilian populations. At the end of 2005, the global figure of "persons of concern" (including refugees, returnees, stateless, and internally displaced persons) stood at 21 million. By the close of 2006, the number stood at 32.9 million, an increase of 56%. At the time of this writing, the estimated number of refugees alone stands at 9.9 million, the highest in 5 years [1].

Each individual refugee has a unique story of development, culture, preflight, flight, and resettlement. Literature shows that refugee populations experience a wide range of stressors such as lack of care, witnessing murders or mass killings, forced labor, lack of food, forced combat, rape, and/or torture [2–4]. Other major experiences include loss or separation of family, friends, culture, and possessions [5–8].

Many reviews and studies have been published on the mental health status of refugees [9–12]. Literature clearly links the stressful experiences of a refugee to increased risk for many mental health issues [13–16]. A large number of studies specifically have measured trauma symptoms, or post-traumatic stress disorder (PTSD), although methods and estimates vary

---

* Corresponding author.
E-mail address: lkmurray@bu.edu (L.K. Murray).

1056-4993/08/$ - see front matter © 2008 Elsevier Inc. All rights reserved.
doi:10.1016/j.chc.2008.02.003

childpsych.theclinics.com

[7,16,17]. Youth refugee populations present with not only PTSD but also with depression, anxiety, and grief issues [6,18–22]. Comorbidity of depression, anxiety, and PTSD is very common [4,23]. The mental health symptoms of young refugees span further to include conduct disorder, social withdrawal, restlessness, irritability, difficulty with relationships, and attention problems [24–26].

In summary, refugee children and adolescents may present with a myriad of symptoms after their traumatic experiences. This diverse clinical presentation requires a treatment model that is able to mitigate a number of internalizing and externalizing symptoms. Refugee populations also require interventions that can adjust to the wide-ranging experiences probably encountered during the phases of preflight, flight, and resettlement.

Considerations in the treatment of refugee youth

In working with populations as complex and varied as refugees, some important considerations are involved around "treatment." First, the unique experiences of refugee populations often put them in need of services on many levels (eg, legal, occupational, educational, social, and individual). Frequently refugee families choose not to seek mental health services until basic needs have been met [27–29]. There is some evidence that immigration stressors or social stressors, such as discrimination, are associated with PTSD symptoms in refugee youth [15,30]. Therefore refugee youth may benefit from multiple levels of services, ideally integrated [31,32]. The focus of this article is on the mental and behavioral health component of services for refugee youth.

Second, it is important to recognize the resiliency of youth. Research clearly demonstrates that not all children who experience trauma, including multiple horrific experiences, show mental health symptoms or problems in functioning [33]. Another proportion of such a population may be mildly symptomatic, perhaps benefiting from support programs or efforts to bolster pre-existing support systems. Finally, a proportion will show significant trauma symptoms and need therapeutic treatment. In this article, which discusses treatment using cognitive behavioral therapy (CBT), the focus is on children experiencing trauma-related symptoms.

Finally, with all clients who have experienced trauma and especially refugee populations, engagement is critical to therapeutic treatment [34–37]. One of the hallmarks of trauma symptomatology is avoidance, which increases the challenges of engagement in therapy and maintaining attendance. In addition, for many refugee youth and families, the process of therapy itself may be alien. Families may have different explanatory models of illness and associated pathways to healing, such as understanding the child's problems in religious, rather than psychologic, terms [38]. Speaking to a relative stranger about personal issues may seem strange and undesirable. Families may be particularly hesitant to talk to a therapist from a different culture or think that using mental health services means they are "crazy." Research suggests that engagement strategies are needed early on and throughout treatment with youth and families and also with key members of the cultural community [38]. Engagement strategies may include making sure practical assistance is offered or that families are linked up with other levels of service, as mentioned previously. Finally, delivering services within service systems that are trusted and accessed by refugee youth, such as school settings, may increase acceptance of and engagement in treatment.

Empirical literature on treatment of refugee youth

The literature on empirically tested mental health treatments of youth refugees is weak [39]. Much of the published material on clinical interventions includes descriptive reports, case studies, or small cohort studies without control groups [40–42]. For example, various holistic or family interventions have been used with refugee populations but are lacking empiric evaluation [28,43–49].

CBT with refugee populations contains some empiric evaluation, much of which is covered in other articles in this issue. For example, Layne and colleagues [50] investigated the use of a school-based trauma- and grief-focused psychotherapy manual with 55 war-exposed Bosnian youth. This and other studies using the same manual (C.M. Layne, W.S. Saltzman, N. Savjak, and colleagues, unpublished manual, 2001) are covered in another article in this issue [51,52]. A different CBT model [53] was used by Ehntholt and colleagues [54] in a controlled study with 26 refugee youth in a school, compared with wait-list control. Another group of researchers has adapted narrative exposure therapy (NET), which is a combination of CBT and testimonial therapy, for youth (KIDNET) [55–57]. Although the empiric evaluation of therapeutic treatments for traumatized refugee youth is limited, studies such as these are showing that CBT-based interventions are promising for refugee populations. This is not to say that other treatments are not effective but rather that CBT interventions currently have the greatest empiric support.

Empirical literature on cognitive behavioral therapy for treatment of child trauma

CBT for PTSD has been evaluated quite extensively in nonrefugee youth [51,58–61] and is considered one of the most efficacious and well-supported interventions for traumatized youth. There has been a growing research literature testing the efficacy of mental health interventions with traumatized child populations, and some recent reviews have examined varying levels of empiric support [33,62–64].

Three individual-focused CBT treatment models for traumatized youth have been evaluated in randomized, controlled trials: trauma-focused CBT (TF-CBT), cognitive-based TF-CBT, and Seeking Safety. TF-CBT has been tested systematically and rigorously by the developers, mainly with sexually abused youth. Various randomized, controlled studies have shown that TF-CBT is superior to treatment-as-usual and to nondirective supportive therapy in reducing PTSD, internalizing and externalizing symptoms, and maintaining these results [65–70]. A multisite randomized, controlled trial with 229 sexually abused children showed statistically significant improvements with TF-CBT in comparison to client-centered therapy [59]. These studies also demonstrated that TF-CBT is effective with other trauma symptoms such as interpersonal trust, perceived credibility, and shame, and that caregivers involved in TF-CBT reported greater improvements in their own mental health. Many of these studies included multiply traumatized children, cross-cultural populations, and children who had complex PTSD. An independent researcher also completed a randomized, controlled trial showing TF-CBT to be superior to a wait-list control condition in improving PTSD and depressive symptoms in sexually abused children [71].

Cognitive-based TF-CBT has been tested in a pilot randomized, controlled trial involving 24 children exposed to single-incident traumatic events [72]. Compared with a wait-list control condition, CBT showed large effect sizes for PTSD, anxiety, and depression. Seeking Safety [73] is a treatment model developed for comorbid PTSD and substance use disorder. It was designed originally for adults and has been evaluated recently in a randomized, controlled trial involving 33 adolescent girls [74]. Compared with treatment-as-usual, those receiving Seeking Safety showed significantly better outcomes in a variety of domains.

Other CBT models for trauma with completed randomized, controlled trials have been developed specifically for school-based work. Cognitive-Behavioral Intervention for Trauma in Schools (CBITS) [75] has been tested using a quasi-experimental design with recent immigrant students and in a randomized, controlled trial with sixth and seventh graders who were exposed to violence, showing significant reductions in PTSD and behavioral symptoms [76,77]. Multimodality Trauma Treatment was shown to decrease trauma-related, depressive, and anxiety symptoms in 14 students [60], and these effects have been replicated in additional studies [78]. The UCLA Trauma/Grief Program was tested on 26 students and showed reductions in PTSD and grief symptoms but not in depression [79]. Classroom-Based Intervention [80] was developed specifically for disasters or ongoing terrorist threat. Preliminary evaluations following an earthquake in Turkey and in the West Bank/Gaza schools and camps for Palestinian refugees have shown improvements on multiple domains [81].

Although these CBT models have the most empiric evidence, there are many other promising treatments for traumatized youth. For example,

Trauma-Systems Therapy is a program that integrates CBT components with services to stabilize the child and/or family environment and to advocate on the child's behalf. An open trial of Trauma-Systems Therapy in 110 children demonstrated significant improvement in PTSD symptoms [82]. Trauma-Systems Therapy has been adapted but not yet evaluated for use with refugee youth.

Empirical literature on treatment for traumatic grief

Critical to refugee populations is the issue of loss and traumatic grief. Most of the treatment models already discussed have integrated components focused on loss, although few have been separately evaluated. TF-CBT [83] has been adapted for use in traumatic grief cases, with some initial data on the distinct effectiveness of the traumatic grief components. The 16-session CBT-child traumatic grief (CTG) model was tested with children 6 to 17 years old who had lost parents or siblings [84]. Results demonstrated that significant improvement in PTSD symptoms and adaptive functioning occurred only during the trauma-focused treatment module (the first eight sessions) of this protocol, whereas CTG improved significantly during both the trauma-focused module and the grief-focused module (the second eight sessions) of the protocol. Another study modified CBT-CTG by decreasing the grief module from eight to four sessions and tested its effectiveness on 39 youth. Results demonstrated that children significantly improved in CTG, PTSD, depression, and anxiety [85]. These two studies, combined with other CTG and adult complicated grief studies [50,86,87], suggest that CTG may be a unique condition consisting of a combination of posttraumatic and unresolved grief symptoms. This literature also suggests that CTG may require sequential trauma- and grief-focused interventions. Because so many refugees are likely to suffer from combinations of trauma and grief, interventions that include both foci may be particularly promising.

Evidence beyond the laboratory

Although many treatments have demonstrable efficacy within randomized, controlled trials, there are far fewer rigorous trials on the delivery of therapies under conditions of routine practice, where issues such as greater diversity of clients, delivery by front-line practitioners or even paraprofessionals, and comorbidity are common [88,89]. The transportability and flexibility of an intervention are important considerations when working with diverse and complex populations. Effectiveness studies have been conducted for some of the interventions mentioned previously. For example, TF-CBT [83] and the Trauma/Grief Program (C.M. Layne, W.S. Saltzman, N. Savjak, and colleagues, unpublished manual, 2001) were used in a large effectiveness study of multiply traumatized and culturally diverse children across nine sites in New York City after the September 11 disaster. Results showed significant improvements in mental health symptomatology [90]. TF-CBT also has been adapted and used with several populations including Hispanics [91], Australians [71], and refugees of African descent [92], with evidence suggesting that TF-CBT maintains its effectiveness with adaptation. Layne and colleagues [50] trained paraprofessionals in Bosnia to implement their Trauma/Grief Program. In addition, the adult version of Seeking Safety has shown successful transportability to diverse cultures including Spanish-speaking adults, female veterans, and prison populations. Such studies suggest that these interventions are adaptable to different cultures, are transportable in regards to training and implementation, and remain effective in less-than-ideal conditions.

Description of cognitive behavioral therapy

Trauma-focused CBT interventions for youth are based on well-established theories and components initially developed for the treatment of fear and anxiety in adults [93,94] and commonly used with traumatized adults [95,96]. Components often are similar to CBT treatments applied to many problems, such as depression and anxiety, in children and adolescents [97–100]. The sharing of components across disorders makes sense, given the myriad of symptoms with which youth who have experienced trauma may present. Although the similarities are many, each evidence-based treatment may have a particular system, order, and application of the components. Because CBT is largely skill-based, components tend to build on one another and help prepare the child for future components.

The acronym "PRACTICE," explained in Box 1, is helpful in listing the components most often seen in CBT models for traumatized youth.

Clinical work with refugees is often done through a phased approach [101] that includes (1) establishing safety and trust, (2) trauma-focused

---

Box 1. The "PRACTICE" acronym for common components of cognitive behavioral therapy for traumatized youth

P – Psychoeducation and parenting skills
R – Relaxation
A – Affective modulation
C – Cognitive processing
T – Trauma narrative
I   – In vivo desensitization
C – Conjoint child/parent sessions
E – Enhancing safety and future skills

treatment, and (3) reintegration. The first phase of establishing safety and trust encompasses the first four components ("PRAC") from the "PRAC-TICE" acronym. In this phase it is not necessary to obtain information about the traumas immediately or to discuss them directly. Refugee youth often assume mistakenly that they should or need to give their trauma stories immediately in treatment. Different models, however, have varying numbers of sessions before exposure or narrative work, some with very few and others with added components such as stabilization.

The following sections briefly review the goals or foci of each component and how they might be implemented with refugee populations based on on-going work with refugee populations (B.H. Ellis, L. Murray, and D. Hunt, personal communication, 2007) [102].

Psychoeducation and parenting skills

Psychoeducation

Some of the first objectives of psychoeducation are to engage, normalize, and validate. With refugee families, it may be helpful to begin by providing information to the family about the role of the therapist and what mental health treatment looks like. Some families may assume that mental health services are reserved for only the severely mentally ill or that the therapist is part of a social services department that may take their child away. In addition, eliciting information from the family about how they understand the child's problems may be useful for planning how to present material in the course of treatment. For instance, the cognitive triad may need to be introduced more slowly and with additional explanation if a family views a child's problems as the result of a spirit jinx and not something that the individual may readily influence or change.

It is important to let refugees and their families understand that widely ranging reactions to stressful experiences are normal. Within some cultures, symptoms may be expressed somatically. It may be helpful to give the youth and caregivers information about some common reactions and to link these reactions to areas of clear value to families. For instance, some families may place less emphasis on children's emotions but may value school success highly. Providing concrete information about how trauma can affect a child's ability to engage in and learn at school may help parents see the value in mental health care.

Another goal of psychoeducation is to instill hope that the patient can feel better. Sometimes it is helpful for a clinician to let the youth know that they have seen other refugees like them improve. A central feature of CBT is safety and building safety skills, with some models integrating this component more extensively [74]. This aspect is woven throughout the treatment components but also should be addressed immediately. For example, refugee youth from different cultures may not be familiar with confidentiality and limits of confidentiality. These considerations should be reviewed and explained as being activated solely as a concern for the patient's safety. Some refugee youth continue to be exposed to trauma, such as neighborhood violence, after resettlement, so it is also essential to assess current safety and to follow up on any immediate safety concerns. It may be important to review general safety issues such as (1) when it is safe to go out in their neighborhood or community, (2) who is a "safe person" in their life right now, and/or (3) a safety plan if they ever feel unsafe.

A final goal of psychoeducation with the TF-CBT model is to present a treatment plan, clearly laying out how many weeks the program will last and what will be done throughout that time. As with most CBT treatments, this plan should convey a spirit of upfront honesty about what the patient will experience during treatment. This aspect is particularly important when working with populations to whom the idea of "therapy" may be quite foreign. Describing a plan and a timeline also helps assure youth and caregivers, takes away any fears of the unknown, and promotes attendance.

The clinical implementation of psychoeducation can vary widely. With some refugee populations, drama or skits may allow the client to demonstrate how they have seen stress reactions expressed in their community [102]. Different techniques work for different individuals, and clinical as well as cultural judgment should be used to decide on the most appropriate technique.

Parenting skills/psychoeducation for caregivers

It is well known that many refugee youth lose their parents, many are orphans, many live with relatives, and some are completely without any caregiver or family. In this respect, it is important to remember many CBT treatments have been shown to be highly effective even without the involvement of a caregiver [50,65,75]. If a caregiver is involved, treatment is explained as a collaborative process in which the caregiver is "the expert on this child." Within some cultures parents may be accustomed to withholding their opinions or ideas out of respect for the professional with whom they are working. CBT treatments view caregivers as central therapeutic agents of change and include them in treatment because they can be a child's strongest source of healing [65,67,69]. This "collaboration" also helps incorporate appropriate cultural issues with which the therapist is unfamiliar. Another goal of psychoeducation is to empower a caregiver to feel capable of providing support for the youth. Communicating to parents that treatment is meant to support the family, and not to undermine parenting practices or authority, is essential.

Often CBT treatments that include caregivers spend some time on parenting skills. The basic goals are to enhance enjoyable caregiver–child interactions and to maximize effective parenting. Before incorporating this component with refugees, it is critical to understand what type of parenting is culturally supported and valued. For example, in the West parents often are taught to "praise" their children for specific behaviors they do well. In other cultures, this behavior may be referred to more softly as "encouragement," or the behaviors that caregivers praise may be different. With caregivers of orphaned refugees, skills may focus on building an attachment with the child. Parenting skills are presented as needed in a family and are incorporated throughout the treatment, rather than devoting multiple full sessions to this component alone.

Relaxation or stress management

The goal of relaxation is to explain the physiologic reactions to stress and to teach techniques to reduce these reactions. People relax in assorted ways, such as taking a walk, talking to a friend, meditating, praying, reading a book, or exercising. It may be necessary to ask children how those around them or in their culture seem to relax. For example, some African populations see traditional dances or singing as relaxing but may not be familiar with meditation. Finally, with refugee youth, it may be important to talk about situations or times when it is appropriate to relax and times that it may not be as safe.

Affective modulation

The first goal of affective modulation is for the clinician to understand the child's vocabulary for different feelings. The child's emotional vocabulary may be shaped by linguistic ability, as in the case of a child who has relatively few emotion words in English but many in his or her own language, or by culture, as in the case of a child whose native language has different means of describing emotions. When there are language barriers, engaging a cultural broker or a bicultural therapist may be important. In addition, drama or making faces that represent certain feelings for the child may help overcome mild language barriers. When culture shapes a child's emotional vocabulary, more extensive care is needed to ensure that therapist and child have a common language. For example, a refugee child may use a local word for a feeling that means "deep within the soul," a word that does not exist in English. As another example, Somali language has relatively few words for emotions but conveys very nuanced emotional experiences through poetry. In these examples the child's emotional vocabulary may be quite rich if the therapist is able to understand how emotions are talked about or communicated in the child's culture. It also is helpful for a clinician to understand the identified feelings from a number of viewpoints, including (1) an example of the situation to which the feeling is linked, (2) where the child might feel a particular emotion in his/her body, and (3) the intensity of a particular feeling word. A clinician also might link identified feelings with another "language" (eg, colors, animals, plants, food, cars, sport). This linking can help if talking about feelings is difficult or when there are language challenges. For example, if traditional dancing or poetry was used in a previous component, a clinician might want to suggest using different dances or poems to represent different feelings.

Cognitive coping skills or the cognitive triad

The first goal of the cognitive coping skills component is to help children distinguish among thoughts, feelings, and behaviors. With refugee youth, it is important first to understand what they think thoughts, feelings, and behaviors are and where in the body thoughts, feelings, and behaviors originate. For example, some children may say thoughts come from the head; others, depending on their cultural background, may say they come from the heart. Some explanatory models may be quite different from the cognitive triad (eg, a child may have been told that his or her behaviors are a result of being jinxed). Some cultures do not draw a distinction between mind and body. Taking a mutually respectful stance and encouraging youth to try out a new way of thinking without undermining cultural beliefs may help in these situations.

The second goal is to help youth make the connection between thoughts, feelings, and behaviors as they relate to everyday life. At first, the situations used should be familiar to the child and should be benign, such as sharing a meal. These goals usually are accomplished by drawing a triangle (Fig. 1), but there are many other creative ways to also achieve these objectives. For example, some refugees may not be familiar with shapes, and a clinician might chose to use a drawing of a body to connect "things that go on in our heads" with "feelings inside us," and "actions that our body does." Once a youth understands the connection, the objectives are to help the patient recognize that negative feelings often originate from inaccurate or unhelpful thoughts [103] and work to view different events in more accurate or helpful ways. Again, these skills should be taught in the context of everyday events and not necessarily around any traumatic experiences. As the child becomes familiar with these skills, they can serve as a tool to work through different crises that may arise between sessions.

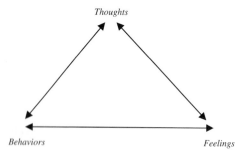

Fig. 1. The cognitive triangle.

Summary of skills

By accomplishing the goals of the first four components ("PRAC"), the clinician has given the youth skills that will be used throughout the creation of the trauma narrative. In addition, the clinician should have learned about the client, including aspects of the client's culture, what relaxation techniques work for the client, how he or she best communicates about emotions, what his or her interests are, what everyday life consists of, and what types of helpful or "unhelpful" cognitions the client may have. Depending on cultural, linguistic, and engagement barriers, accomplishing the "PRAC" goals may take more time for some children than others. Especially when refugees have been deliberately harmed by authority figures, establishing trust with a therapist who holds a position of relative power may take extra time. For refugee youth, moving to the trauma narrative portion of treatment should take place only after the necessary skills and trust are in place. When done in a culturally sensitive manner, the components of PRAC can be a remarkable way to bond and build trust with someone while simultaneously teaching skills.

Trauma narrative

Directly talking about the trauma is a technique that some avoid when working with traumatized children. One reason for this avoidance may be caregiver or youth discomfort in talking about the trauma. Others may be nervous about "pushing the child," or further traumatizing the child. Most CBT interventions developed for youth conceptualize the trauma narrative as a slow process in which the clinician is more of a guide, allowing the unspeakable to be spoken. Contrary to a belief that telling the narrative may further traumatize a youth, it actually allows a child to gain mastery over trauma reminders or triggers, to resolve avoidance symptoms, and to correct distorted or unhelpful cognitions. Extensive literature demonstrates that exposure treatment is effective with a variety of anxiety-related treatment [59,95,104].

The trauma narrative usually is created in the form of a book but can also be expressed in other creative ways such as a poem, song, dance, interview, or computer presentation. For refugee populations that are likely to have experienced a host of traumatic experiences, completing a timeline is helpful. The timeline gives the child an opportunity to write down any experiences he or she believes are important and gives the clinician some perspective on how the youth views those experiences. For each event, a chapter or section may be written. Sections may be about an event (eg, "village invasion"), a time of chronic trauma (eg, "when the rebels kept coming"), important cultural omissions (eg, "the death ceremony that never happened"), or even ongoing instability within resettlement periods (eg, "my first day in the new place," "the second foster home"). In this way, children are not required to identify a single "worst" event. With each chapter or section, clinicians start the child at a specific point in time to help the client walk through the trauma in a step-wise fashion, with more and more details given. As the story is gone over repeatedly, the child slowly becomes desensitized to the material.

A critical part of the trauma narrative is the cognitive reprocessing work. Once a traumatic event is written about, the clinician asks the youth about thoughts and feelings he or she had at the different points. In this way, it becomes clear where different maladaptive, inaccurate, or unhelpful cognitions may lie. Cognitive restructuring techniques are used to help the child come to a more helpful thought, potentially leading to different (more positive) emotions and behaviors. The trauma narrative is finalized with a section on what the child learned, what he or she might want to tell other refugee children, or how the client is different now.

If a caregiver is involved in a refugee child's treatment, ideally the trauma narrative would be shared with the caregiver after each session. In this way, a caregiver also is desensitized slowly to the material in the book and also understands more about the thoughts and feelings related to the events. The sharing of the trauma narrative is important so that the child has someone in his or her life who has heard the story and with whom the child is comfortable sharing openly. Often entire refugee families have shared traumatic experiences. Some parents may not be ready to hear their child's narrative, especially if it describes their own traumatic experiences as well. As with the child, the parent needs to have acquired the skills and established the trust necessary to be a part of sharing the trauma narrative.

In vivo desensitization

In vivo desensitization may not be needed in all cases. If the feared situation or place is distant or the traumatizing stimuli are not accessible, this process may not be possible. There may be situations in which this component, whose goals are to desensitize the child to trauma reminders and resolve avoidance, may be used.

Conjoint parent-child sessions

As described previously, care must be taken not to share a child's trauma narrative without first ensuring that the caregiver is adequately prepared. If a caregiver is involved and capable of being supportive to the child, there is a joint session to share the trauma narrative. The goals include sharing the trauma narrative, opening communication between caregiver and child, and furthering cognitive reprocessing. For refugee children who may be without a caregiver, this session may be done with any adult with whom the youth is connected (eg, a case-worker, legal aid, camp leader, or teacher).

Enhancing safety skills

Enhancing safety skills is a large component of many CBT trauma programs and occurs throughout the treatment, with the overall goal of preparing for future trauma reminders or safety situations. With refugee populations, this component may include developing safety plans for any of a variety of situations they fear may occur. This component also could entail skills training on other issues such as healthy sexuality, bullying behavior, problem-solving skills, or interpersonal communication skills. Youth who have spent a great deal of their childhood in refugee camps may have developed ways of relating interpersonally that are inappropriate in other cultures, such as using aggression to get one's needs met. Focusing on social or healthy living skills may be an important way to increase safety and also to provide assistance with non–trauma-related emotional and behavioral needs of refugee youth. Often youth are encouraged to return to their timeline and extend it to the future. This component shares some of the objectives of the final phase commonly used in refugee work, or reintegration.

Components for addressing childhood traumatic grief

In cases of traumatic grief, the "PRACTICE" components often help a child become "unstuck" from trauma symptoms, opening the client up to a more healthy grieving process. The first CTG component is grief psychoeducation. With refugee youth, it is essential to understand how death and mourning are understood by them and their native culture. For example, a clinician might ask the youth to draw a picture of what he or she thinks happens when someone dies [105]. In addition, the clinician should focus on understanding grief reactions the child may be experiencing.

The second component includes grieving or reminiscing about the loss of the deceased or missing, considering both the experiences the child had with that person in the past and the experiences they might have shared in the future. For example, a clinician might ask the child to identify, name, act out, or draw the things he or she did with the deceased or missing person. For refugee children this process may contain mundane situations, rituals, or meaningful places. Talking about the future helps prepare a child for reminders of loss when the deceased or missing person is not present for events and enables the client to create a coping plan (C.M. Layne, W.S. Saltzman, N. Savjak, and colleagues, unpublished manual, 2001). Another goal often includes resolving ambivalent feelings about the deceased or missing person. For example, some refugee youth may have been separated from a loved one suddenly and unexpectedly, with no time for "good-byes." This abrupt separation may lead to lack of resolution, guilty feelings, resentment, or anger that a child may feel cannot be voiced. A clinician might use the skills taught within the "PRACTICE" components to restructure some thoughts, encourage a child to have a "mental conversation" with the deceased or missing person or the person's spirit, or to write a letter to the absent person. The goal with refugees would be to guide them through a meaningful and culturally appropriate way of honoring the deceased or missing person and sending that person on.

Additional components help the child shift to the positive and focus on the future. For example, a child may be encouraged to think of positive memories of the deceased or missing person. Some children may put together a memory box or a collage with positive experiences or things about the deceased or missing person. For refugee children, it may be helpful to hold a memorial ceremony for the deceased, especially if there is some cultural ritual that they feel was absent. To focus on the future, a child is encouraged to redefine the relationship with the deceased or missing person and commit to present relationships. With refugees, activities may be used to talk about what they are missing and what they still have in the present. It is particularly important that refugee children be given skills to feel that it is acceptable to move on to other relationships so a support system can be established in the current culture. These two components attempt to address reintegration issues further, similar to a phased approach commonly advocated with refugee populations.

Additional considerations

A number of other considerations should be addressed when working with refugee populations. For example, a clinician often must work through an interpreter because of language barriers. CBT manuals usually are well laid out so translators can become familiar with some of the session material in advance. In some cases, especially when whole communities have been traumatized, participating in the trauma narrative may be emotionally difficult for interpreters. Providing additional training and debriefing for interpreters may be helpful. In some circumstances a cultural brokering model can be developed. Another consideration is that some refugees may not have attended school and thus present with lower cognitive development and often do not have skills such as writing, reading, and drawing. CBT interventions designed for youth (eg, activities done in dramatic rather than written form) are adapted easily to these situations. Another common issue, particularly when working abroad with refugee populations, is the advantage of working in groups (C.M. Layne, W.S. Saltzman, N. Savjak, and colleagues, unpublished manual, 2001) [75]. The model can incorporate moving through the components (particularly the first four "PRAC" components) with multiple youth. Depending on the experiences and safety levels, the trauma narrative sessions might be completed individually.

Summary and future directions

There is a vast literature base showing that refugee youth are likely to encounter numerous and varied traumatic events that can have widely devastating and long-term effects in a range of areas. The resulting symptoms and child/family circumstances are equally diverse, making treatment challenging at best. The empiric evaluation of mental health treatments with refugee youth is increasing but remains weak. The available research with nonrefugee populations suggests that CBT is highly efficacious in treating traumatized youth and the complex myriad of symptoms with which they present. Current efforts are focused on extending these empirically sound treatments into the mainstream, testing their ability to perform under more naturalistic conditions and with culturally diverse populations. Some CBT interventions already have shown significant results with refugee youth populations [50,54,57]. It is likely that many of the CBT treatments rigorously tested with nonrefugee youth (eg, TF-CBT, CBITS) could produce similar reductions in the diverse emotional, cognitive, and behavioral symptoms presented by traumatized refugee youth.

CBT has certain characteristics that may be particularly advantageous in the treatment of refugee youth. For example, CBT treatments are skill-based with the goal of giving children and families the abilities to work through issues beyond the treatment. CBT is theoretically grounded in what has been demonstrated to be effective for trauma symptomatology including its diversity and comorbidity. CBT also is time-limited, increasing the chances for sustainability and commitment from clients. Finally, certain CBT interventions have demonstrated flexibility in how goals are implemented, opening many opportunities for cross-cultural modifications while maintaining fidelity.

The current state of literature on treatment for traumatized youth suggests that the time is ripe to move beyond counting those affected and describing their problems and into evaluating the effectiveness of interventions with young refugees. Overall, there are many promising interventions for refugee youth that could use empiric evaluation and empirically supported interventions for traumatized youth that could be adapted for and disseminated to refugee populations. It will be important to evaluate empirically interventions with children who may be at varying levels of ongoing risk, such as children who have relocated to a safe area versus those who may remain within a camp and/or in a tumultuous zone. For those working with refugee populations who have relocated to Europe or the United States, studies of how cultural adaptations increase acceptance of and engagement in treatment within refugee communities and of the effectiveness of these treatments in improving functioning and the ability to take advantage of other services would be advantageous. For researchers working with young refugee populations in low-resource countries, it will be important to examine the training process, the acceptability of the intervention to the local culture, its cost effectiveness, and its sustainability. Finally, in both countries of resettlement and refugee camps, investigating how CBT and trauma processing can best be integrated with other services and needs could enhance greatly the overall system of care for refugee youth. Although the understanding of how to treat refugee youth effectively is advancing, much work remains to be done.

References

[1] United Nations High Ccommissioner for Refugees. Available at: http://www.unhcr.org/statistics/STATISTICS/4676a71d4.pdf. Accessed November, 2007.

[2] Boothby N. Trauma and violence among refugee children. In: Marsella A, Bornemann S, Ekblad J, et al, editors. Amidst peril and pain: the mental heath and well-being of the world's refugees. Washington, DC: American Psychological Association; 1994.

[3] Fox PG, Cowell JM, Montgomery A. Southeast Asian refugee children: violence experience and depression. Int J Psychiatr Nurs Res 1996;5:589–600.

[4] Kinzie JD, Sack WH, Angell RH, et al. The psychiatric effects of massive trauma on Cambodian children, I: the children. J Am Acad Child Adolesc Psychiatry 1986;25: 370–6.

[5] Berry JW. Refugee adaptation in settlement countries: an overview with an emphasis on primary prevention. In: Ahearn FL, Athey JL, editors. Refugee children: theory, research and services. Baltimore (MD): Johns Hopkins University Press; 1991. p. 20–38.

[6] Eisenbruch M. From post-traumatic stress disorder to cultural bereavement: diagnosis of Southeast Asian refugees. Soc Sci Med 1991;33:673–80.

[7] Rothe E, Lewis J, Castillo-Matos H, et al. Posttraumatic stress disorder among Cuban children and adolescents after release from a refugee camp. Psychiatr Serv 2002;53:970–6.

[8] Tobin JJ, Friedman J. Intercultural and developmental stresses confronting Southeast Asian refugee adolescents. Journal of Operational Psychiatry 1984;15:39–45.

[9] Jensen PS, Shaw J. Children as victims of war: current knowledge and future research needs. J Am Acad Child Adolesc Psychiatry 1993;32:697–708.

[10] Keyes EF. Mental health status in refugees: an integrative review of current research. Issues Ment Health Nurs 2000;21:397–410.

[11] Lustig SL, Kia-Keating M, Knight WG, et al. Review of child and adolescent refugee mental health 1993. J Am Acad Child Adolesc Psychiatry 2004;43(1):24–36.

[12] Rousseau C. The mental health of refugee children. Transcultural Psychiatric Research Review 1995;32:299–331.

[13] Athey JL, Ahearn FL. The mental health of refugee children: an overview. In: Athey JL, editor. Refugee children: theory, research, and services. Baltimore (MD): Johns Hopkins University Press; 1991. p. 3–19.

[14] Almqvist K, Broberg AG. Mental health and social adjustment in young refugee children 31/2 years after their arrival in Sweden. J Am Acad Child Adolesc Psychiatry 1999;38: 723–30.

[15] Sack WH, Clarke GN, Seeley J. Multiple forms of stress in Cambodian adolescent refugees. Child Dev 1996;67:107–16.

[16] Steele Z, Silove D, Bird K, et al. Pathways from war trauma to posttraumatic stress symptoms among Tamil asylum seekers, refugees, and immigrants. J Trauma Stress 1999;12:421–35.

[17] Kinzie JD, Boehnlein JK, Leung PK, et al. The prevalence of posttraumatic stress disorder and its clinical significance among Southeast Asian refugees. Am J Psychiatry 1990;147: 913–7.

[18] Papageorgiou V, Frangou-Garunovic A, Iordanidou R, et al. War trauma and psychopathology in Bosnian refugee children. Eur Child Adolesc Psychiatry 2000;9:84–90.

[19] Servan-Schreiber D, Lin BL, Birmaher B. Prevalence of posttraumatic stress disorder and major depressive disorder in Tibetan refugee children. J Am Acad Child Adolesc Psychiatry 1998;37:874–9.

[20] Felsman JK, Leong FTL, Johnson MC, et al. Estimates of psychological distress among Vietnamese refugees: adolescents, unaccompanied minors and young adults. Soc Sci Med 1990;31:1251–6.

[21] Nader K, Pynoos RS, Fairbanks L, et al. A preliminary study of PTSD and grief among the children of Kuwait following the Gulf crisis. Br J Clin Psychol 1993;32:407–16.

[22] Smith P, Perrin S, Yule W, et al. War exposure among children from Bosnia-Hercegovina: psychological adjustment in a community sample. J Trauma Stress 2002;15:147–56.

[23] Sack WH, McSharry S, Clarke GN, et al. The Khmer adolescent project. I. Epidemiological findings in two generations of Cambodian refugees. J Nerv Ment Dis 1994;182:387–95.

[24] Mollica RF, Poole C, Son L, et al. Effects of war trauma on Cambodian refugee adolescents' functional health and mental health status. J Am Acad Child Adolesc Psychiatry 1997;36:1098–106.

[25] Almqvist K, Brandell-Forsberg M. Refugee children in Sweden: post-traumatic stress disorder in Iranian preschool children exposed to organized violence. Child Abuse Negl 1997; 21:351–66.

[26] Tousignant M, Habimana E, Biron C, et al. The Quebec Adolescent Refugee Project: psychopathology and family variables in a sample from 35 nations. J Am Acad Child Adolesc Psychiatry 1999;38:1426–32.

[27] Geltman PL, Augustyn M, Barnett ED, et al. War trauma experience and behavioral screening of Bosnian refugee children resettled in Massachusetts. J Dev Behav Pediatr 2000;21:255–61.

[28] Sveaass N, Reichelt S. Refugee families in therapy: from referrals to therapeutic conversations. Journal of Family Therapy 2001;23:119–35.

[29] Watters C. Emerging paradigms in the mental health care of refugees. Soc Sci Med 2001;52: 1709–18.

[30] Ellis BH, McDonald H, Lincoln A, et al. Mental health of Somali adolescent refugees: the role of trauma, stress, and perceived discrimination. J Consult Clin Psychol, in press.

[31] Papadopoulos R. Working with Bosnian medical evacuees and their families: therapeutic dilemmas. Clin Child Psychol Psychiatry 1999;4:107–20.

[32] Ellis BH, Rubin A, Betancourt TS, et al. Mental health interventions for children affected by war or terrorism. Chapter 7. In: Feerick M, Silverman G, editors. Children exposed to violence. Baltimore, MD: Brookes Publishers; 2006.

[33] Finkelhor D, Berliner L. Research on the treatment of sexually abused children: a review and recommendations. J Am Acad Child Adolesc Psychiatry 1995;34:1408–23.

[34] McKay M, McCadam K, Gonzales J. Addressing the barriers to mental health services for inner-city children and their caretakers. Community Ment Health J 1996;32(4):353–61.

[35] McKay M, Nudelman R, McCadam K. Involving inner-city families in mental health services: first interview engagement skills. Res Social Work Pract 1996;6:462–72.

[36] McKay M, Stoewe J, McCadam K, et al. Increasing access to child mental health services for urban children and their care givers. Health Soc Work 1998;23:9–15.

[37] McKay MM, Hibbert R, Hoagwood K, et al. Integrating evidence-based engagement strategies into "real-world" child mental health settings. Brief Treatment and Crisis Intervention 2004;4:177–86.

[38] Ellis BH. Somali adolescents and pathways to mental health care: understanding help seeking within one refugee community. Presented at the 23rd Annual Meeting of the International Society for Traumatic Stress Studies, Baltimore, MD, November 15–17, 2007.

[39] Feldman R. Primary health care for refugees and asylum seekers: a review of the literature and a framework for services. Public Health 2006;120:809–16.

[40] Basoglu M. Behavioural and cognitive treatment of survivors of torture. In: Jaranson JM, Popkin MK, editors. Caring for victims of torture. Washington, DC: American Psychiatric Press; 1998. p. 131–48.

[41] Moore LJ, Boehnlein JK. Posttraumatic stress disorder, depression and somatic symptoms in U.S. Mien patients. J Nerv Ment Dis 1991;179:728–33.

[42] Morris P, Silove D, Manicavasagar V, et al. Variations in therapeutic interventions for Cambodian and Chilean refugee survivors of torture and trauma: a pilot study. Aust N Z J Psychiatry 1993;27:429–35.

[43] Aroche J, Coello M. Towards a systematic approach for the treatment rehabilitation of torture and trauma survivors in exile: the experience of STARTTS in Australia. Presented at

the 4th International Conference of Centres, Institutions and Individuals Concerned with Victims of Organized Violence: "Caring for and Empowering Victims of Human Rights Violations", DAP, Tagaytay City, Philippines, December 5–9, 1994. Available at: http://www.startts.org.au. Accessed November, 2007.

[44] Papadopoulos RK. Refugee families: issues of systemic supervision. Journal of Family Therapy 2001;23:405–22.

[45] Arrendondo P, Orjuela E, Moore L. Family therapy with Central American war refugee families. Journal of Strategic and Systemic Therapies 1989;8:28–35.

[46] Bemak F. Cross-cultural family therapy with Southeast Asian refugees. Journal of Strategic and Systemic Therapies 1989;8:22–7.

[47] Mehraby N. Therapy with refugee children. Available at: http://www.swsahs.nsw.gov.au/areaser/Startts/article_2.htm. Accessed November, 2007.

[48] Silove D, Manicavasagar V, Beltran R, et al. Satisfaction of Vietnamese patients and their families with refugee and mainstream mental health services. Psychiatr Serv 1997;48:1064–9.

[49] Woodcock J. Healing rituals with families in exile. Journal of Family Therapy 1995;17:397–409.

[50] Layne CM, Pynoos RS, Saltzman WS, et al. Trauma/grief focused group psychotherapy: school based post-war intervention with traumatized Bosnian adolescents. Group Dynamics 2001;5:277–90.

[51] Goenjian AK, Karayan I, Pynoos RS, et al. Outcome of psychotherapy among early adolescents after trauma. Am J Psychiatry 1997;154:536–42.

[52] Goenjian AK, Walling D, Steinberg AM, et al. A prospective study of posttraumatic stress and depressive reactions among treated and untreated adolescents 5 years after a catastrophic disaster. Am J Psychiatry 2005;162:2302–8.

[53] Smith P, Dyregrov A, Yule W, et al. Children and war: teaching recovery techniques. Bergen (Norway): Foundation for Children and War; 2000. Available at: http://www.childrenandwar.org. Accessed May 15, 2007.

[54] Ehntholt KA, Smith PA, Yule W. School-based cognitive-behavioural therapy group intervention for refugee children who have experienced war-related trauma. Clin Child Psychol Psychiatry 2005;10:235–50.

[55] Onyut LP, Neuner F, Schauer E, et al. Narrative exposure therapy as a treatment for child war survivors with posttraumatic stress disorder: two case reports and a pilot study in an African settlement. BMC Psychiatry 2005;5:1–9.

[56] Schauer E, Neuner F, Elbert T, et al. Narrative exposure therapy in children: a case study. Intervention 2004;2:18–32.

[57] Ruf M, Schauer M, Neuner F, et al. KIDNET—a highly effective treatment approach for traumatized refugee children. Paper presented at the European Conference on Traumatic Stress (ECOTS). Opatja, Croatia, June 5–9, 2007.

[58] American Academy of Child and Adolescent Psychiatry. Practice parameters for the assessment and treatment of children and adolescents with posttraumatic stress disorder. J Am Acad Child Adolesc Psychiatry 1998;37:4S–26S.

[59] Cohen JA, Deblinger E, Mannarino AP, et al. A multisite randomized controlled trial for children with sexual abuse-related PTSD symptoms. J Am Acad Child Adolesc Psychiatry 2004;43:393–402.

[60] March JS, Amaya-Jackson L, Murray MC, et al. A cognitive-behavioral psychotherapy for children and adolescents with posttraumatic stress disorder after a single-incident stressor. J Am Acad Child Adolesc Psychiatry 1998;37:585–93.

[61] Saigh PA. The use of an in vitro flooding package in the treatment of traumatized adolescents. J Dev Behav Pediatr 1989;19:17–21.

[62] Cohen JA, Berliner L, March JS. Treatment of children and adolescents. In: Foa EB, Keane TM, Friedman MJ, editors. Effective treatments for PTSD: practice guidelines from the International Society for Traumatic Stress Studies. New York: Guilford Press; 2000. p. 106–38, 330–2.

[63] Chorpita BF. Toward large-scale implementation of empirically supported treatments for children: a review and observations by the Hawaii Empirical Basis to Services Task Force. Clinical Psychology: Science and Practice 2002;9:165–90.

[64] Saunders BE, Berliner L, Hanson RF, editors. Child Physical and Sexual Abuse: Guidelines for Treatment (Final Report: January 15, 2003). Charleston. SC: National Crime Victims Research and Treatment Center; 2003.

[65] Deblinger E, Lippmann J, Steer R. Sexually abused children suffering posttraumatic stress symptoms: initial treatment outcome findings. Child Maltreat 1996;1:310–21.

[66] Deblinger E, Steer RA, Lippman J. Two-year follow-up study of cognitive-behavioral therapy for sexually abused children suffering posttraumatic stress symptoms. Child Abuse Negl 1999;23:1371–8.

[67] Cohen JA, Mannarino AP. A treatment outcome study for sexually abused preschool children: initial findings. J Am Acad Child Adolesc Psychiatry 1996;35:42–50.

[68] Cohen JA, Mannarino AP. Interventions for sexually abused children: initial treatment findings. Child Maltreatment 1998;3:17–26.

[69] Cohen JA, Mannarino AP. A treatment outcome study for sexually abused preschool children: outcome during one-year follow-up. J Am Acad Child Adolesc Psychiatry 1997;36(9):1228–35.

[70] Cohen JA, Mannarino AP, Knudson K. Treating sexually abused children: 1 year follow up of a randomized controlled trial. Child Abuse Negl 2005;29:135–45.

[71] King NJ, Tonge BJ, Mullen P. Treating sexually abused children with posttraumatic stress symptoms: a randomized clinical trial. J Am Acad Child Adolesc Psychiatry 2000;39:1347–55.

[72] Smith P, Yule W, Perrin S, et al. Cognitive behavior therapy for PTSD in children and adolescents: a preliminary randomized controlled trial. J Am Acad Child Adolesc Psychiatry 2007;46:1051–61.

[73] Najavits LM. Seeking safety: a treatment manual for PTSD and substance abuse. New York: Guilford Press; 2002.

[74] Najavits LM, Gallop RJ, Weiss RD. Seeking safety therapy for adolescent girls with PTSD and substance use disorder: a randomized controlled trial. J Behav Health Serv Res 2006; 33:453–63. Available at: www.seekingsafety.org. Accessed October, 2007.

[75] Jaycox LH. Cognitive-behavioral intervention for trauma in schools. Longmont (CO): Sopris West Educational Services; 2003.

[76] Kataoka SH, Stein BD, Jaycox LH, et al. A school-based mental health program for traumatized Latino immigrant children. J Am Acad Child Adolesc Psychiatry 2003; 42(3):311–8.

[77] Stein BD, Jaycox LH, Kataoka SH, et al. A mental health intervention for schoolchildren exposed to violence: a randomized controlled trial. JAMA 2003;290(5):603–11.

[78] Amaya-Jackson L, Reynolds V, Murray MC, et al. Cognitive-behavioral treatment for pediatric posttraumatic stress disorder: protocol and application in school and community settings. Cogn Behav Pract 2003;10(3):204–13.

[79] Saltzman WR, Pynoos RS, Layne CM, et al. Trauma- and grief-focused intervention for adolescents exposed to community violence: results of a school-based screening and group treatment protocol. Group Dynamics: Theory, Research and Practice 2001;5:291–303.

[80] Macy RD. Community-based trauma response for youth. New Dir Youth Dev 2003;(98): 29–49.

[81] Khamis V, Macy R, Coignez V. Impact of the classroom/community/camp-based intervention program on Palestinian children: US Agency for International Development and SAVE report on Palestinian children. Available at: http://www.usaid.gov/wbg/reports/Save2004_ENG.pdf. 2004.

[82] Saxe GN, Ellis H, Fogler J, et al. Comprehensive care for traumatized children: an open trial examines treatment using trauma system therapy. Psychiatr Ann 2005;53:443–8.

[83] Cohen JA, Mannarino AP, Deblinger E. Treating trauma and traumatic grief in children and adolescents. New York: Guildford Press; 2006.

[84] Cohen JA, Mannarino AP, Knudsen K. Treating childhood traumatic grief: a pilot study. J Am Acad Child Adolesc Psychiatry 2004;43:1225–33.

[85] Cohen JA, Mannarino AP, Staron VR. A pilot study of modified cognitive-behavioral therapy for childhood traumatic grief (CBT-CTG). J Am Acad Child Adolesc Psychiatry 2006;45:1465–73.

[86] Prigerson HG, Shear MK, Rank E, et al. Traumatic grief: a case of loss-induced trauma. Am J Psychiatry 1997;154(7):1003–9.

[87] Prigerson HG, Shear MK, Jacobs SC. Consensus criteria for traumatic grief: a preliminary empirical test. Br J Psychiatry 1999;174:67–73.

[88] Hoagwood KE, Burns BJ, Kiser L, et al. Evidence-based practice in child and adolescent mental health services. Psychiatr Serv 2001;52(9):1179–89.

[89] Chorpita BF. Treatment manuals for the real world: where do we build them? Clinical Psychology Science and Practice 2002;9:431–3.

[90] Final report on the Child and Adolescent Trauma Treatment Consortium (CATS) project for the Substance Abuse and Mental Health Services Administration (SAMHSA). October 2006. Substance Abuse and Mental Health Services Administration. Available at: www.samhsa.gov.

[91] de Arellano MA, Danielson CK. Culturally-modified trauma-focused therapy for treatment of Hispanic child trauma victims. Presented at the Annual San Diego Conference on Child and Family Maltreatment. San Diego, CA; January 22–26, 2006.

[92] Center for Multicultural Human Services. Member of the National Child Traumatic Stress Network. Available at: www.nctsn.org. Accessed November, 2007.

[93] Wolpe J. Basic principles and practices of behavior therapy of neuroses. Am J Psychiatry 1969;125(9):1242–7.

[94] Beck AT. Cognitive therapy and the emotional disorders. Oxford (UK): International Universities Press; 1976.

[95] Foa EB, Rothbaum BO, Riggs DS, et al. Treatment of post-traumatic stress disorder in rape victims: a comparison between cognitive-behavioral procedures and counseling. J Consult Clin Psychol 1991;59:715–23.

[96] Keane TM, Fairbanks JA, Caddell JM, et al. Implosive (flooding) therapy reduces symptoms of PTSD in Vietnam combat veterans. Behav Ther 1989;20:245–60.

[97] Kazdin AE, Weisz JR. Evidence-based psychotherapies for children and adolescents. New York: Guilford Press; 2003.

[98] Weisz JR, Hawley KM, Doss A. Empirically tested psychotherapies for youth internalizing and externalizing problems and disorders. Child Adolesc Psychiatr Clin N Am 2004;13(4): 729–815, Special issue: Evidence-Based Practice, Part I: Research Update.

[99] Kazdin AE, Weisz JR. Identifying and developing empirically supported child and adolescent treatments. J Consult Clin Psychol 1998;66:19–36.

[100] Ollendick TH, King NJ. Empirically supported treatments for children and adolescents. In: Kendall PC, editor. Child and adolescent therapy: cognitive—behavioral procedures. New York: Guilford Press; 2000. p. 386–425.

[101] Herman JL. Trauma and recovery from domestic abuse to political terror. New York: Basic Books; 1997.

[102] Stepakoff S, Hubbard J, Katoh M, et al. Trauma healing in refugee camps in Guinea: a psychosocial program for Liberian and Sierra Leonean survivors of torture and war. Am Psychol 2006;61:921–32.

[103] Seligman MEP, Reivich K, Jaycox L, et al. The optimistic child. Boston: Houghton, Mifflin and Company; 1995.

[104] Keane TM, Marshall AD, Taft CT. Posttraumatic stress disorder: etiology, epidemiology, and treatment outcome. Annu Rev Clin Psychol 2006;2:161–97.

[105] Stubenbort KJ, Donnelly GR, Cohen J. Cognitive-behavioral group therapy for bereaved adults and children following an air disaster. Group Dynamics: Theory, Research and Practice 2001;5:261–76.

ELSEVIER
SAUNDERS

Child Adolesc Psychiatric Clin N Am
17 (2008) 605–624

CHILD AND
ADOLESCENT
PSYCHIATRIC CLINICS
OF NORTH AMERICA

Group Interpersonal Psychotherapy for Depressed Youth in IDP Camps in Northern Uganda: Adaptation and Training

Helen Verdeli, PhD[a,b,c,*],
Kathleen Clougherty, MSW[b,c], Grace Onyango, MA[d],
Eric Lewandowski, MSc[a], Liesbeth Speelman, MA[e],
Teresa S. Betancourt, ScD[f],
Richard Neugebauer, PhD[b,c], Traci R. Stein, MPH[a],
Paul Bolton, MBBS[g]

[a]Teachers College, Columbia University, Box 102, 525 West 120th Street, New York,
NY 10027, USA
[b]New York State Psychiatric Institute, Columbia University, 1051 Riverside Drive,
Unit 24, New York, NY 10032, USA
[c]College of Physicians and Surgeons, Columbia University, 1051 Riverside Drive,
Unit 24, New York, NY 10032, USA
[d]World Vision Uganda, P.O. Box 5319, Plot 15B, Nakasero Road, Kampala, Uganda
[e]War Child Holland, Gulu, Uganda
[f]Harvard University School of Public Health, 651 Huntington Avenue, 7th floor,
Boston, MA 02115, USA
[g]Johns Hopkins Bloomberg School of Public Health, 615 N Wolfe Street,
Room E8646, Baltimore, MD 21205, USA

This article reviews the use of interpersonal therapy in a specific population of displaced children, and describes and discusses the methods used to adapt interpersonal therapy for this population. Armed conflicts expose children to prolonged and repeated stressors that can have severe immediate and long-term psychologic consequences, including posttraumatic stress (PTSD), depression, and behavioral and conduct problems [1–3]. Additionally, the emotional and cognitive development of young children may be

* Corresponding author. Teachers College, Columbia University, Box 102, 525 west 120th street, New York, NY 10027.
  E-mail address: hv2009@columbia.edu (H. Verdeli).

1056-4993/08/$ - see front matter © 2008 Elsevier Inc. All rights reserved.
doi:10.1016/j.chc.2008.03.002
childpsych.theclinics.com

affected by constant fear; severe losses or disruptions in relationships with caregivers, family, and community members; limited access to formal education; exposure to malnutrition and infections; and pressure to prematurely assume adult family roles [4,5].

Among a sample of 61 Tibetan child and adolescent refugees living in India, 11.5% were found to meet DSM-IV criteria for PTSD and 11.5% for major depressive disorder [6]. A well-known longitudinal study of 40 Cambodian refugees resettled in the United States found a 50% prevalence of PTSD and 56% prevalence of depression 4 years after leaving refugee camps in their home country [7]. Nine years after the first study, depression rates were 14% and PTSD rates were 35% [8].

In a sample of 229 Palestinian children and adolescents exposed to violence since the start of the Second Uprising, almost 70% were identified as having PTSD and 40% as having moderate to severe depression. Additionally, 70% showed poor coping responses [9]. Other studies that did not report on posttraumatic stress symptoms have identified depression and internalizing behaviors in children in response to war-related trauma. For example, exposure to war stress was related to internalizing symptoms in 121 children from Gaza aged 6 to 16 years [10].

A study of Bosnian children and adolescents showed the highest rates of depressive symptoms in children whose father had disappeared during the war and whose current whereabouts were unknown. These children exhibited even more depression than those whose fathers had disappeared and were eventually confirmed dead [11]. Despite variability in the relative prevalence of depression and PTSD and differences in their duration after exposure to war stress, both seem highly prevalent adverse mental health outcomes in children and adolescents exposed to war and dislocation.

An exponential growth in studies of youth afflicted by war and violence occurred over the past 2 decades, indicating the increased attention devoted to mental health problems by the international humanitarian community. However, most of these studies use Western instruments to measure mental health outcomes in non-Western resource-poor communities without first validating these instruments locally. Similarly, mental health interventions for humanitarian emergencies have been increasingly included in the global health agenda, resulting in the fielding of various treatment programs. These interventions have been developed mostly in Western countries, based on Western assumptions about human relationships, communication, and coping.

Although the value of some interventions has been rigorously tested in Europe or the United States, assessments in other settings are rare. Thus, discrimination among helpful, ineffective, and harmful interventions for resource-poor areas in non-Western countries is exceedingly difficult given the paucity of evidence on their efficacy in these settings [12]. The lack of scientific evidence on programs addressing the psychologic needs of war-affected adolescents is especially pronounced [13].

To fill this scientific and programmatic gap, a research collaboration among three groups was formed in 2004: Bolton and colleagues from Boston University (BU); two Interpersonal Psychotherapy experts from Teachers College and the New York State Psychiatric Institute, College of Physicians and Surgeons, Columbia University; and two non-governmental organizations (NGOs): World Vision and War Child Holland (WCH). This two-step research program had the goal of selecting mental health problems in the youth important for the local population and potentially amenable to interventions; and assessing in a randomized clinical trial (RCT) the impact of the mental health interventions on these problems [14,15].

Previously, the three collaborating groups conducted a RCT with depressed adults in Southern Uganda. In that study, group interpersonal psychotherapy (IPT-G) showed efficacy for treating depression with some anxiety symptoms in adults. Compared with an assessment-only control group, IPT-G led to significantly higher symptom and functional improvement, with results persisting in the 6-month follow-up [16,17]. However, because the control condition included no intervention, the question remained whether the specific IPT-G skills or a more general nonspecific group-support effect was operative.

A second condition, a form of creative play therapy developed by WCH was included. IPT-G and creative play therapy were compared with a wait-list control group.

The Awer and Unyama camps in the northern province of Gulu were selected for study because they represent the service catchment area of the two NGO partners. Awer camp is located southwest from Gulu town, with a population of approximately 27,000. The camp has little legal economic activity, such as shops or businesses. Unyama camp, with a population of 20,000, is closer to Gulu and somewhat more economically active than Awer. Residents of Awer and Unyama have attempted small-scale farming near the camps, because it is considered too dangerous to farm farther afield (Paul Bolton, MBBS, and colleagues, World Vision Internal Report, 2006).

Armed conflict in Northern Uganda

The 20-year-old armed conflict in Northern Uganda between the rebel Lord's Resistance Army (LRA) and the Ugandan government is among the deadliest humanitarian emergencies in the world. The LRA has committed countless atrocities against Ugandan civilians from the northern Acholi ethnic group, including rape, mutilation, and murder.

One of the LRA's most notorious crimes against humanity involves the abduction of more than 25,000 children to serve as soldiers and labor/sex slaves. Abductees habitually witnessed and were victims of horrific acts of violence, such as severe beatings, marching until exhaustion, rape, and mutilation. Captive children were occasionally forced to kill others, including relatives and friends [18].

Internally displaced persons camps in Northern Uganda

This conflict has displaced 1.8 million Ugandans to internally displaced persons (IDP) camps guarded by the Ugandan military. Most of this population has been exposed to significant psychologic trauma. A survey among adults at an IDP camp in Pader found that 79% of respondents had witnessed torture and 40% a killing. Of respondents, 63% reported the disappearance/abduction of a family member and 58% had lost a family member to violence.

This survey also found that men and women experienced the local syndrome "par," which shares many symptoms with major depressive disorder, including low mood, sadness, poor appetite, sleep disruption, social withdrawal, and thoughts of suicide. Women were considerably more likely to experience Par than men. Suicidal thoughts in the week before the survey were reported by 63% of women and 13% of men. All respondents could identify one person who had attempted suicide in the past month. Men and women also reported current symptoms of traumatic stress [19].

In these camps, the normal fabric of society has been eroded by dislocation, fear, and death from violence and disease. Traditional social structures have been disrupted and the routines of life and education of youth suspended. Women fear rape and abduction and bear the burden of caring for their family without the traditional support of kin and community elders. Men have lost their traditional role as the family provider. Because finding work is difficult and dangerous, camp residents are often idle and become dependent on humanitarian programs. Fear and hopelessness contributes to high rates of alcohol abuse and domestic violence, and hunger drives women of all ages to prostitute themselves. Little is known specifically about the impact of the conflict on the mental health of children and adolescents (Paul Bolton, MBBS, and colleagues, World Vision Internal Report, 2006) [20].

Preintervention assessment

In July 2004, the BU team initiated a two-step assessment process, a qualitative followed by a quantitative study. The assessment was conducted in Luo, the local language. The qualitative study identified (1) major mental health and psychosocial issues affecting the camp youth, as experienced and perceived by the local community; and (2) youth tasks and activities that the community considered important, such as the ability to perform gender-specific chores, attend school, interact with peers, and fulfill family and community roles. This information was then used to inform the design of quantitative instruments of mental health problems and associated dysfunction. These instruments were then used to assess the impact of candidate mental health interventions in the RCT [14,15].

The results of this assessment have been described in detail elsewhere [14]. In summary, the qualitative study yielded seven locally described syndromes. Two states of mind—a legitimate fear of LRA attacks and "cen," an agitated posttraumatic stress reaction experienced by local people as attack by evil spirits seeking revenge—were determined by the BU and NGO research team as unlikely to be amenable to psychosocial intervention with available resources.

Three of the remaining local syndromes (two tam, par, and kumu) were local depression-like problems with mixed depression and anxiety symptoms. The fourth (ma lwor) was an anxiety-like local syndrome, and the fifth (kwo maraco) involved a combination of conduct problems. Alcohol abuse and sexual violence were part of several of these syndromes [14,15].

A locally derived quantitative instrument was developed, the Acholi Psychosocial Assessment Instrument (APAI), to incorporate the symptoms of the five major syndromes and a measure of functional limitations experienced during the past week. The APAI depression scale contained all symptoms of the depression-like syndromes. A cut-off score on the APAI depression scale was determined based on discrimination of cases versus noncases. Reliability and validity are discussed in works by Bolton and colleagues [14] and Betancourt [15].

Randomized clinical trial

Participants

The RCT by Bolton and colleagues [14] screened 667 youth, with 314 adolescents aged 14 to 17 years meeting inclusion criteria. Study inclusion criteria included residence in the camps in the month preceding the screening interview, depression-like symptoms for at least 1 month and currently exceeding the predetermined cutoff score, functional impairment, and assent (adolescents) and consent (caregivers).

Exclusion criteria were severe cognitive or physical disability that would impair ability to answer questions in Luo, and active/persistent suicidal ideation/behavior. Posttraumatic and other anxiety symptoms and substance use problems were not exclusionary criteria. A total of 304 participants who met inclusion criteria agreed to take part in the study; 57% were girls and 42% had been previously abducted by the LRA [14]. The study was sanctioned by local community leaders.

Interventions

The results of the qualitative and quantitative study showed that depression-like syndromes were both prominent and debilitating in adolescents in these camps; among those assessed, 45% were met inclusion criteria. However, the local depression-like syndromes contained a high number of anxiety symptoms. Comorbid anxiety in depressed adolescents is routinely encountered in Western countries (rates ranging from 15%–60%) [21,22] and, given the degree of danger and trauma in the lives of the camp population, was expected to be at least as high in the current sample.

When making decisions about candidate interventions addressing depression or trauma/anxiety, the authors decided to include IPT-G for several reasons. First, during the qualitative study, youth and caregivers reported that their main concerns revolved around daily life in the camps, including struggles for survival and access to food and education. Negotiation of space (given the overcrowding in the camps), the readjustment of abducted youth to the camp life, and dealing with the burden of caretaking of members of their family of origin and new family were some prominent issues for adolescents. Adult caregivers also complained that the adolescents were disrespectful and unmotivated.

Furthermore, United States studies indicate that IPT for depressed adolescents who had comorbid anxiety had positive effects on depression and comorbid anxiety. Among 48 adolescents aged 12 to 18 years diagnosed with major depression, those who participated in IPT treatment experienced greater reductions in depressive symptoms and more improvement in social and global functioning than those who underwent clinical monitoring [23].

A study of adolescents aged 12 to 17 years experiencing various depressive disorders found that IPT was significantly more effective in reducing symptoms of depression than usual treatment. This study also showed that the presence of comorbid anxiety symptoms did not diminish the effectiveness of IPT-A, which continued to be superior to usual treatment, and was in fact associated with a near-significant increase in the effectiveness of IPT-A relative to usual treatment [24].

Lastly, IPT-G has shown efficacy for treating depression with some anxiety symptoms in adults in South Uganda. Compared with an assessment-only control group in an RCT, IPT-G led to significantly higher symptom and functional improvement, with results persisting in the 6-month follow-up [16,17].

The partner NGO World Vision and local communities adopted and disseminated the treatment, which is still practiced by the original clinicians and has been administered to approximately 2500 community members (Grace Onyango, MA, personal communication, 2007). A main reason for selecting IPT-G for South Uganda was its compatibility with the cultural attitude of experiencing self as an integral part of a social and ethnic group. This attitude also characterizes the Acholi population in Northern Uganda.

Interpersonal psychotherapy for groups

IPT was originally developed in the United States as an individual treatment for unipolar nonpsychotic depression [25]. In treating depression, IPT targets the connection between onset of symptoms and current interpersonal problems. IPT therapists begin with a systematic diagnostic assessment, explain the diagnosis, and work with the patient to identify the problem areas associated with the onset of current symptoms.

Difficulties in four interpersonal areas are considered triggers of depressive episodes and become the focus of treatment: (1) grief (from death of a loved one), (2) interpersonal disputes (disagreements with important people in one's life), (3) role transitions (negative and positive changes in life circumstances), and (4) deficits (persistent problems in initiating or sustaining relationships) [26].

IPT is specified in a manual, has been tested in numerous open and randomized clinical trials, and is efficacious for several mood and non–mood disorders among adolescent, adult, and geriatric outpatient populations [26]. The feasibility and efficacy of individual IPT for treating symptoms of depression in adolescents in clinical settings has been tested in open, randomized, controlled clinical trials [23,27]. Its effectiveness in treating depression in adolescents recruited and treated in school-based clinics by community mental health professionals was subsequently established [28]. IPT for depressed adolescents (IPT-A) typically consists of 12 weekly sessions and has the goal of decreasing depressive symptoms and improving interpersonal functioning. As with IPT for adults, IPT-A conceptualizes interpersonal difficulties as fitting into one or more of the four problem areas mentioned earlier [23].

IPT was adapted for groups (IPT-G) and was found to be efficacious in treating binge-eating disorder [29], postpartum depression [30], and depressed adults in communities in South Uganda [16,31]. IPT-A has also been adapted for use as a 12-session group intervention [32]. A group therapy context can provide adolescents with additional peer support and opportunities to practice interpersonal skills.

The adaptation of IPT-G for South Uganda specified one or two pre–group meetings, which are individual meetings between the leader and each group member followed by 16 weekly group meetings lasting 90 minutes (Kathleen Clougherty, MSW, and colleagues, unpublished manual, 2002).

In IPT-G, members are encouraged to practice new communication and interpersonal problem-solving skills in the group. They inform each other about progress in their weekly goals. Therapists also make supportive and cohesion-building process remarks.

Termination is the fourth phase of treatment, with particular emphasis on enhancing each patient's independent functioning and developing strategies for relapse prevention. It usually lasts 2 to 4 sessions in IPT and IPT-G clinical trials.

Creative play

Creative play was developed by WCH to promote social skills, self-esteem, and self- expression for war-affected children [33]. It typically lasts 12 weeks and is provided to children aged 6 to 14 years in their communities, and is based on the premise that their coping will be strengthened by verbal and nonverbal expression of thoughts and feelings through age-appropriate creative activities, such as singing, art, role-playing, and music. [33]. The content of the group meetings is not fixed and is usually organized around themes relevant to the children's circumstances. For example, if the goal is to build trust among peers, then facilitators might encourage a collaborative game in which each child leans on the others with eyes closed, supported entirely by the rest of the children.

For the RCT, creative play was used with children aged 14 to 17 years diagnosed with depression-like illnesses, and extended to 16 weekly sessions of 1.5 to 2 hours. The games and exercises were adapted for this age group. The groups of 11 to 25 adolescents were of mixed gender, and were facilitated by two WCH social workers (one man and one woman). Its adaptation for Northern Uganda focused on integrating formerly abducted and nonabducted children, thus facilitating social cohesion.

Activities drawn from the WCH manuals were adapted for developmental level by the local facilitators and supervisors, and included games, drama, songs, art, and debates. Weekly sessions began with warm-up exercises followed by focused group activities. Groups ended with a closing activity, such as a game and an opportunity for participants to provide feedback on how they felt about that day's activities.

Although some WCH programs have incorporated therapy-based elements into their postactivity discussions, this study declined to use this strategy to more clearly delineate the contrast between the IPT-G and creative play. Although participants in crisis could discuss problems with creative play facilitators after group meetings, this was not typical and only occurred on a few occasions (eg, with a young woman whose baby had just died, and a formerly abducted boy who was overwhelmed by memories of his life with the rebels). The two facilitators were supervised on a weekly or bimonthly basis by the WCH Psychosocial Specialist, who discussed the program and shared reports regularly with the BU staff through email and weekly phone conversations.

Creative play had several features that rendered it an ideal comparison group to IPT-G. The group format controlled for nonspecific group effects, such as hope, group member support, attention by members and facilitator, reduction of social isolation, and structure of time (an important element in the IDP camps). In addition, some important antidepressant skills, common to effective treatments of depression [34], were operative in creative play, such as behavioral activation (increase in pleasurable and mastery activities) and social skills building.

Creative play also had significant credibility in the community because its facilitators had strong ties with the camp youth and had earned the confidence and respect of the community. Finally, from the beginning of the study, the facilitators believed that creative play would lead to significant clinical and functional improvement, paralleling the IPT-G facilitator expectations.

Wait-list controls

During the study period, participants in the control group received no intervention. However, they could access services and programs not linked to the study. The adolescents who were assigned to the control condition, along with their caregivers, were informed at the beginning of the study that if they agreed to participate, they would be first to receive either (or both) CP or IPT-G intervention, which were shown to be effective at reducing the depression-like symptoms that were the target of the RCT.

Development of group interpersonal psychotherapy for depression in Northern Uganda

Two IPT experts of the research group undertook the manual adaptation for this project and the training and supervision of the group leaders. Before the visit to the site they prepared a draft of the manual based on the IPT-G manual from Southern Uganda, and hypothesized that some basic assumptions of the IPT-G model would at least be somewhat relevant to the Northern Ugandan youth [31].

The first of these assumptions was that three of the four interpersonal problem areas of IPT (grief, interpersonal disputes, and role transitions) would be triggers of depression in the camp youth, similar to those in Southern Uganda. The authors were unsure whether the fourth IPT problem area, interpersonal deficits, would be a relevant trigger for depression. To determine if it would be pertinent in communities, they planned to ask the trainees open-ended nonleading questions about what made local youth depressed, and then judge whether their responses corresponded to the four problem area.

The second assumption was that strengthening interpersonal skills would improve depression. Offering an opportunity to mourn losses while receiving group support; building skills to contain grief; improving communication and decision-making regarding relationships, roles, and readjustments; and assisting youth to support each other would result in symptomatic improvement. Evidence for this has been shown in several clinical trials in Western countries and in the RCT in Southern Uganda. However, the authors had misgivings about whether the skills that IPT-G offered were potent enough to protect the adolescents against these extreme adversities.

Adapting the manual

In May 2005, the IPT trainer traveled to the Gulu district to train prospective group leaders who were fluent in English and Luo; training was conducted in English. The main source of information about the local culture was the trainee group members, because they lived in the districts participating in the study. In addition, Bolton and colleagues, who had conducted the qualitative study, consulted with the team on a regular basis. The Southern Uganda IPT-G manual was adapted on-site for cultural relevance (Kathleen Clougherty, MSW, and colleagues, unpublished manual, 2002). Its language was free of jargon (ie, grief was called *death of a loved one*; disputes were *disagreements*; transitions were *changes*; and interpersonal deficits were *loneliness and shyness*) and included detailed scripts in simple language with numerous clinical examples. This section discusses adaptations made in consultation with trainee group leaders.

Developmental adaptations

Developmental issues characteristic of adolescence were considered in this adaptation. The first was the necessity for involvement of caregivers in the therapy. The leader met separately with a caregiver in at least the initial pre–group sessions and for a termination session either with or without the adolescent. The second were the frequent and abrupt changes of mental status and high reactivity among adolescents. The leaders were instructed to monitor very closely symptom changes and emergence of suicidality, which was rampant in the camps.

Finally, the adaptation considered the multiple roles and issues these adolescents had, some typical of adolescence (eg, disagreements with caregivers about going out with friends, disrespectful behavior), and some characteristic of young adults (eg, caring for other children, either their own or siblings; taking financial responsibility for themselves and often the family; having to pay for secondary school education).

Diagnosing depression

In IPT, diagnosis of depression occurs during the initial meeting between the group leader and each group member individually. Therapists begin by diagnosing depression and clarifying its triggers and treatment. During training, the trainees were asked to describe adolescents with the three depression-like syndromes and discuss the behavior and community reaction. It was emphasized that the group leader had to convey to the adolescents that they are not "mad," and offer hope by saying that this condition is treatable.

The assignment of the "sick role" presented a challenge, because lowering expectations about optimal performance and functioning when these adolescents were struggling for survival was frequently unrealistic; not fetching clean water or being late for food distribution had serious life-or-death consequences. The facilitators believed that educating adolescents and caregivers about the impact of depression on functioning, offering hope and support, and removing the guilt and blame about suboptimal performance had important impacts on adolescents. However, the trainees supported the right of the caregivers to insist on being respected.

Explaining the treatment contract

Role of the leader

During the initial pre–group meeting, the leader's task was to explain to the adolescent and caregiver and how the group would proceed. Like in Southern Uganda, the leaders emphasized to the adolescents repeatedly during the group meetings that they would not provide material goods (the community was used to World Vision and other NGOs providing financial and health-related benefits). Instead, leaders explained that they and the group members would be supporting each other to determine what situations contribute to depression and what can be done about the situations to feel better. The leaders also explained that they could all work together to find ways to identify people in the community, government, and NGOs who could provide financial and medical assistance on an ongoing basis, and persuade them to help.

Confidentiality and trust

The group members were asked not to disclose the content of the group meetings to people outside the group. Although no major instances of breach of confidentiality were raised, the leaders reported to their supervisors another, deeper problem during the trial: they felt that initially, the adolescents showed a significant lack of trust, and frequently refrained from revealing specifics about their life circumstances (either not giving an accurate account or withholding information). It was not unusual for adolescents to open up during the second half of the treatment (after session 8).

For example, one girl who had been living with her "uncle" eventually revealed in the ninth session that he was a man with whom she had eloped. A boy eventually revealed that the death of his brother was not caused by a snake bite but from suicide. Through supervision and self-reflection, the leaders understood these reactions as the adolescents' need for self-protection, and supported and celebrated with the rest of the group each adolescent's decision to open up.

One technique that many leaders found useful was to talk in the beginning of the session about general issues that that camp adolescents frequently confronted (eg, pregnancy, substance use, suicidality, domestic violence, abductions) without referring to specific individuals, and discuss what IPT skills might help manage these issues. Leaders found this helped adolescents reveal more personal material. For example, one leader knew that a young woman was not discussing her unwanted pregnancy. When arriving early for a session once, the leader found many used condoms strewn about an area in the camp. She took this opportunity to discuss sexual behavior and condom use. A large outdoor celebration had occurred the previous night, and as the group talked about what happens at these parties, the adolescent who had previously avoided group discussions opened up and began sharing with the group.

Flexibility

Sixteen weekly sessions at a specific place within the camps (eg, community center, church, open space) were initially planned. However, the trainees cautioned that significant flexibility had to be built into the structure to make the project viable. For example, adolescents frequently came late or skipped sessions during planting season, food distribution, hospitalization of self or family member, and major camp events.

For safety reasons, leaders could only work in the camps during the day, which made it difficult to find a weekday time for the groups to meet because many adolescents attended school. Most group meetings were switched to meet on Saturdays. In the first couple of sessions, several adolescents did not attend the session, either because of work or shyness. The leaders sought them out and reported that by the third session the adolescents started attending regularly. Sometimes the leaders needed to ease the way for adolescents to attend the group by asking parents and caregivers to allow their children to perform chores at other times.

Problem areas

When asked about triggers of depression in these communities, the trainees identified interpersonal problems that corresponded with all four IPT problem areas (death of a loved one, disagreements, life changes, and social isolation). Contrary to the trainees in South Uganda, these felt that social isolation was not just an epiphenomenon of a life change, but a problem on its own. The facilitators in this project found that several adolescents, mostly abductees, had significant gaps in their interpersonal skills because they spent critical periods of their development in the bush. For instance, the use of language was minimal in captivity because whistling and clapping formed the bush vocabulary. These gaps resulted in isolation and social deficits when the children returned to the IDP community. The following examples, presented during supervision, were characteristic illustrations of problem areas and peculiarities in their presentations because of camp circumstances.

Death of a loved one

Adolescents often encountered the death of a family member or friend from violence (which adolescents occasionally witnessed either first-hand or second-hand through its impact on the dead in the aftermath) or illness, including AIDS, malnutrition, accidents. As in South Uganda, when dealing with traumatic loss, facilitators asked the adolescents for details about what was witnessed, addressing the last time the adolescent saw the loved one alive and what happened during that time; helped adolescents to remember and mourn the relationship with the deceased; and supported the adolescent's new ties to other people. Adolescents were then asked what they wished they had said or done at that time. The grieving adolescents were invited to bring items that reminded them of the loved ones.

Those frequently overwhelmed by thoughts about the deceased were instructed to put some time aside during the day to think about their loved ones, while trying to retain focus on other activities during the rest of the day. Occasionally, family members had been abducted and the adolescent did not know whether they were dead or alive. The leaders conceptualized these incidents as transition problems, helping adolescents focus on how hope or despair affects them, helping them refocus their energy on self-improvement and -care and care of other loved ones.

Disagreements

Adolescents argued with caregivers about issues such as the latter's expectation for the adolescents, including being more involved in the household, contributing to the family income, protecting the family honor, and being more respectful. Many disagreements (overt or covert, such as silent marginalization) occurred with relatives other than parents who had to care for the adolescent after parental death. These caregivers often had different expectations about the role the adolescent would play in their lives. Rampant substance use by the adults and occasionally the youth fuelled these arguments.

Sometimes the disagreements occurred among children; for example, siblings or neighbors fighting about access to resources. As with IPT in South Uganda, the authors helped adolescents develop communication skills, focusing on how to convey a point without necessarily being direct, because Western-like directness would often cause worse problems for the adolescent.

Using culturally appropriate options when resolving a dispute was an important goal. Some options considered useful and adaptive in that culture would not be considered as such in the West. For instance, the group frequently suggested that, when fighting with caregivers, adolescents not answer back and ignore them, which worked surprisingly well. Another strategy was to find powerful advocates who could influence the other person. For example, a boy whose father disagreed with his decision to go to school was encouraged by the group to talk to his uncle, who had influence over the father and could make him change his mind. Furthermore, a girl who had disagreements with her father because he would not let her practice traditional dance talked to the father's relatives who persuaded him to be more lenient.

Life changes

Life changes included returning to the camp after being abducted, having a new family (numerous adolescents considered themselves married, and some had or were expecting children), taking care of the family of origin (usually because of parental death), becoming sick with AIDS and other illnesses, and being unable to find work to pay school fees. The challenge was to identify and focus on the elements that the individual could control and work on skill-building and identification of options.

Facilitators noted that depression makes individuals feel more powerless than they are in reality, and helping them explore various options is worthwhile instead of assuming a priori that these are unrealistic or will be unsuccessful. For example, a boy who was significantly burdened because he had to care for his infant sister after their parents' death was encouraged to identify relatives who could care for her.

Another powerful tool incorporated into the work was helping adolescents find advocates with power who could assist them, while also learning skills to communicate effectively with that person. The group members happily exchanged information about matters such as how to apply for school fees and identify NGOs and other resources to improve their condition.

Although the groups were usually very supportive of members, especially to abducted boys who opened up about their experiences, occasionally they were less accepting of particular life transitions. Some girls complained that when they were abducted life was easier for them. One 15-year-old girl who was a rebel commander's wife during her abduction described the beautiful clothes her husband brought her and how she was never hungry then. When she lamented her loss of privilege, the group was restrained and numb in their responses to her.

Social isolation

The authors found only four cases of social isolation, always as a secondary problem area to a life change or death of a loved one. Emphasis was placed on building skills for the life change while helping the individuals break the social isolation. For example, a 17-year-old girl who cried frequently in the group was very lonely after the death of her parents, with whom she was close. She had trouble hearing, and other children teased her "because (she) looked like a boy." The leader and group helped her mourn, supported her, and discussed ways to respond to those who teased her and seek out more understanding companions.

Case example

A is a 16-year-old depressed girl living in an IDP camp in northern Uganda. She is an orphan with no history of abduction whose parents were killed by the rebels 5 years ago. At the time of the group, *A* was living with her grandmother. Her problem areas, which were determined during the two pre-group meetings, included life change because of her current pregnancy and frequent disagreements with her abusive, blind grandmother who felt that *A* no longer listened or helped at home. *A*'s long-term goals were to find a way to earn a living so that she could take care of herself and her baby, and to reduce the arguments with and abuse by her grandmother.

A was active during the initial phase of the group, discussing her disagreements with her grandmother and her need to prepare for her baby's arrival. The group was helpful in suggesting how she could cope better with her grandmother (eg, ignore and avoid) and supporting her ideas for earning a living. However, approximately halfway through the treatment, A disclosed that the father of her baby abandoned her on discovering she was pregnant. By the end of the group, A was earning a living through farming and selling her produce, and had worked out many problems with her grandmother through a combination of doing more of what her grandmother wanted and following the group's suggestion to ignore the grandmother and avoid engaging in arguments.

When these methods were not possible, the group suggested that she cook bad food for her grandmother. As a result, the grandmother became alarmed by the change in A's behavior and questioned her. A told her grandmother how the beatings made her feel, and the grandmother was able to admit her fear that A would abandon her. At a follow-up visit, the therapist learned that A had delivered a healthy baby, whom her grandmother caring for while A worked. Disagreements at home were significantly reduced and A's mood had significantly improved.

Special clinical issues during the trial

The following clinical vignettes show the importance of careful monitoring and planning to manage adverse events when conducting trials of this nature.

Cen

G was a 17-year-old boy randomized to the IPT-G condition who had been abducted by LRA rebels twice and forced to kill people, including his brother-in-law's brother. G had previously experienced episodes of cen ("being haunted by the spirits of those that one killed") before participating in the trial. During the middle phase of IPT-G, his cen attacks re-emerged. During treatment, his wife was expecting a child and he heard that the wife of the man he had killed intended to bring her 5 children to him so he could care for them.

While G was participating actively and opening up in the IPT-G treatment group, on two successive occasions he experienced blackouts or a period of brief psychosis or dissociation, and injured himself. He described being outside with friends when a "spirit" attacked him. He started shouting and friends brought him to his house and locked the door, after which he started hitting the walls. He hit the walls of his hut hard enough to break bones in his hands and hit his knees with a hammer, causing swelling. A similar event occurred a few days later.

These two episodes occurred around the time he began to talk in the IPT group about his history of being abducted as a child soldier and forced to kill others. Per the IRB plan, this young man was assessed by the lead psychosocial advisor for the NGO War Child Holland in North Uganda.

The clinician who evaluated G did not believe that his living environment in the camp was safe enough to contain his symptoms at that time. He was placed at the World Vision Rehabilitation center (one of the two NGO part-ners involved in the study) for formerly abducted children to be stabilized. Because he was a formerly abducted child, the NGO World Vision paid for his hand surgery (from the injuries sustained during his blackout), and the hospital fees for his wife's delivery. He was suspended from group participa-tion for three sessions during his surgery. Given his connection to the IPT-G group, both *G* and his facilitator (who saw him as a leader in the group) were upset by the suspension and viewed it as punishment. The authors had to conduct additional individual supervision with the group facilitator, who had come to lean heavily on *G* in the group given his comfort with disclosing his experiences and his ability to provide support to others in the group. The facilitator had several anxieties that his group would be unsuccessful without *G* involved.

Once it was evident that *G* was more stable and was receiving support from individual and family counseling in the interim care center, he was al-lowed to return to the group. *G* was able to attend the last IPT-G sessions, but he and many others in his group lamented the period he had been away.

Suicidal group

The group of six suicidal adolescents who were excluded from the study met weekly, a male and female facilitator were assigned to lead the group, and the facilitators were encouraged to make mid-week individual visits to anyone deemed to require more clinical monitoring. Except for closer monitoring, the flow of the suicidal group mirrored that of the traditional IPT groups. At termination the group members improved significantly and no suicide attempts were made during the trial.

M is an example of a typical adolescent from this group. She reported that the trigger for her grief was the recent death of her husband, who had been killed in an ambush by the LRA. Through the first eight sessions, she used the group to mourn the loss of her husband. In session nine she finally revealed that her grief was caused by the multiple deaths in her immediate family and the death of her husband by suicide, not murder.

She described in detail her husband's suicidal ideations, his behavior on the day of his death, his method of suicide, and the events after his death, including the burial. The group comforted *M*, told her that she was not alone, and suggested she be strong for her young sick child. The facilitators observed that *M*'s mood had improved. Her hygiene also improved and she became more talkative, reported feeling better, and concluded that the group was a place where people would listen to her. After the group, *M* started attending literacy classes.

Training

IPT-G training took place on-site in northern Uganda over 13 days. Twelve trainees (six men and six women) attended. All were familiar with the camps and lived in nearby communities. Each trainee either had or was working toward a college degree and had work experience with children (eg, teaching, youth team leadership). Training was conducted in English, and all trainees were proficient in English and Luo.

The training was developed by two senior Columbia IPT consultants and was implemented on-site by one these consultants and three World Vision staff, two of whom were clinicians in the original IPT-G southwest Uganda trial and the third was an experienced psychosocial trainer. The authors used a combination of didactics and experiential methods to teach basic IPT group principles and techniques. They treated the training group as an experiential group to show the trainees the development of group dynamics and processes.

The first goal of the training was to make the trainees comfortable working in a group. The trainers began by talking about themselves and their work, and sharing some personal information. The trainees were then asked to do the same. When this activity was completed, the trainees were asked to reflect on how it felt to talk about themselves among strangers. Some described feeling embarrassed, anxious, and worried about being judged. One trainee disclosed a personal history of abduction. Their experiences of the activity were used to explore what group members might feel when they first join an IPT group.

Next the training was divided into four phases to reflect the pre-group, initial, middle, and termination phases of group IPT. IPT-G skills characteristic of the pre–group phase include learning to talk to group members, forming a therapeutic alliance, expressing empathy, assessing depression symptoms, taking a relevant history, conducting the interpersonal inventory, establishing the problem area and setting related goals, psychoeducation about depression, explaining IPT-G treatment (including confidentiality), and obtaining consent from the patient to join the group. The authors expanded the knowledge the trainees had from earlier work with adolescents to establish basic guidelines on how to communicate with that age group. Next, pre–group tasks were broken down as outlined earlier and each component systematically taught.

In this type of training, trainers demonstrate IPT concepts in front of the class, followed by break-out groups of initially two and then three trainees. The practice occurs first in English so the trainers can listen and know what the trainees have learned, and then in Luo so the trainees become comfortable with what they will actually say when they are with the adolescents. This approach, including repetition in both languages, is key to training inexperienced or less-experienced clinicians in a brief timeframe.

The authors asked trainees to practice each section of IPT pre–group in the evening, because the amount of work that could be done in the evenings was limited as the trainees lived at home during these 2 weeks. The authors' recommendation for future trainings is that all participants stay together for the training period. The goal is always to have trainees become familiar enough with the concepts and scripts that they do not need to rely on notes.

To learn the phases of IPT-G, the trainees needed to learn to conduct group therapy and understand the IPT concepts and techniques. During these phases, the trainees learned to assess patient mood and symptoms during a group; encourage members to disclose within a group; link mood change to events; mobilize the group members to support each other and make suggestions; and encourage members to try out new approaches for improving their interpersonal problems.

The final phase of training is intended to mirror the termination phase of IPT-G. Trainees were taught the tasks they needed to learn during this phase, and were encouraged to draw from their experience in ending their training to understand a group's potential feelings about finishing IPT-G.

Results of the clinical trial

Results, presented in detail by Bolton and colleagues [14], showed that although all three groups (IPT-G, CP, and WLC) showed decline in mean depression symptom scores between baseline and termination, mean depression symptom scores in the IPT-G were significantly lower than in the WLC group. Among girls, IPT-G was superior to WLC in reducing depression symptom scores. Boys' results, although in the expected direction, were not statistically significant. Creative play showed no effect on depression severity scores. Neither IPT-G nor creative play was associated with significant improvement in anxiety or conduct-like syndrome scores in the total sample. Also, neither treatment group showed improvement in functioning or conduct problems.

Preliminary analyses showed that a history of abduction was associated with higher baseline depression scores, although this factor did not affect the change within any of the three study groups at termination.

Summary

The authors adapted IPT-G for this population knowing that IPT was a good fit for depressed Ugandan adults. However, they questioned whether it would be effective for depressed Ugandan adolescents dealing with extreme adversity. Research findings from Southern Uganda and two subsequent years of IPT groups in that region showed the usefulness and transportability of this Western psychotherapy. The four IPT problem areas resonated with this population as triggers for depression: death of a loved one, life changes, disagreements with important persons, and, to a lesser degree, loneliness and social isolation. The "here and now" focus was appropriate in this adolescent population, for whom solving current problems was often essential to survival, and relying on others for support and help was culturally compatible.

The authors understand that they are far from proclaiming that this approach "cured" depression and its associated disability in this population. Although IPT-G significantly lowered depression in girls, it did not significantly impact depression in boys, nor did it affect the functioning of both boys and girls. Speculations about its lack of effectiveness in those targets and suggestions for improvement have been presented elsewhere [14].

In the scope of this article, IPT-G proved to be feasible in its training and implementation, was accepted as a treatment option by the community, and, to an important extent, reduced depression significantly for several adolescents. The control group has been treated with IPT-G, as promised, and the group leaders are currently treating depressed adolescents in eight IDP camps in Northern Uganda, showing the sustainability and adoptability of the IPT-G program (Grace Onyango, MA, personal communication, 2007).

References

[1] Brajsa-Zganec A. The long-term effects of war experiences on children's depression in the Republic of Croatia. Child Abuse Negl 2005;29:31–43.

[2] Barenbaum J, Ruchkin V, Schwab-Stone MS. The psychosocial aspects of adolescents exposed to war: practice and policy initiatives. J Child Psychol Psychiatry 2004;45(1):41–62.

[3] Derluyn I, Broekaert E, Schuyten G, et al. Post-traumatic stress in former Ugandan child soldiers. Lancet 2004;363(9412):861–3.

[4] Lasser J, Adams K. The effects of war on children: school psychologist's role and function. Sch Psychol Int 2007;28(1):5–10.

[5] Srour RW, Srour A. Communal and familial war-related stress factors: the case of the Palestinian child. Journal of Loss and Trauma 2006;11:289–309.

[6] Servan-Schreiber D, Lin B, Birhamer B. Prevalence of post-traumatic stress disorder and major depressive disorder in Tibetan refugee children. J Am Acad Child Adolesc Psychiatry 1998;37(8):874–9.

[7] Kinzie JD, Sack WH, Angell RH, et al. The psychiatric effects of massive trauma on Cambodian children: I. The children. J Am Acad Child Psychiatry 1986;25:370–6.

[8] Sack WH, Him C, Dickason D. Twelve-year follow-up study of Khmer youths who suffered massive war trauma as children. J Am Acad Child Adolesc Psychiatry 1999;38(9):1173–9.

[9] Elbedour S, Onwuegbuzie AJ, Ghanna J, et al. Post-traumatic stress disorder, depression, and anxiety among Gaza Strip adolescents in the wake of the second Uprising (Intifada). Child Abuse Negl 2007;31(7):719–29.

[10] Qouta S, Punamaki RL, El Sarraj E. Mother-child expression of psychological distress in war trauma. Clin Child Psychol Psychiatry 2005;10(2):135–56.

[11] Zvizdic S, Butollo W. War-related loss of one's father and persistent depressive reactions in early adolescents. European Psychologist 2000;5(3):204–14.

[12] Bolton P, Betancourt TS. Mental health in postwar Afghanistan. JAMA 2004;292(5):626–8.

[13] Mohlen H, Parzer P, Resch F, et al. Psychosocial support for war-traumatized child and adolescent refugees: evaluation of a short-term treatment program. Aust N Z J Psychiatry 2005;39(1–2):81–7.

[14] Bolton P, Bass J, Betancourt T, et al. Interventions for depression symptoms among adolescent survivors of war and displacement in northern Uganda: a randomized controlled trial. JAMA 2007;298(5):519–27.

[15] Betancourt T. A qualitative study of psychosocial problems war-affected youth in Northern Uganda. Journal of Transcultural Psychiatry, in press.

[16] Bolton P, Bass J, Neugebauer R, et al. A clinical trial of group interpersonal psychotherapy for depression in rural Uganda. JAMA 2003;289:3117–24.

[17] Bass J, Neugebauer R, Clougherty KF, et al. Group interpersonal psychotherapy for depression in rural Uganda: 6-month outcomes—randomised controlled trial. Br J Psychiatry 2006;188:567–73.

[18] Coalition to Stop the Use of Child Soldiers. Child soldiers global report 2004. Available at: http://www.reliefweb.int/rw/lib.nsf/db900SID/LHON66UJKU/$FILE/child_soldiers_CSCnov_2004.pdf?OpenElement. Accessed February 2, 2008.

[19] Medecins Sans Frontieres (2004) Pader: a community in crisis. Available at: http://www.msf.org/msfinternational/invoke.cfm?objectid=CD3DA72E-43DE-4DF5A2BFDA6C49D620F1&component=toolkit.pressrelease&method=full_html. November 8. Accessed February 2, 2008.

[20] Uganda Conflict Action Network (2008). Available at: www.ugandacan.org. Accessed February 11, 2008.

[21] Goodman R, Ford T, Simmons H, et al. Using the strengths and difficulties questionnaire (SDQ) to screen for child psychiatric disorders in a community sample. Int Rev Psychiatry 2003;15:166–72.

[22] TADS Team. Fluoxetin, CBT and their combination for adolescents with depression. JAMA 2004;292(7)):807–20.

[23] Mufson L, Weissman MM, Moreau D, et al. Efficacy of interpersonal psychotherapy for depressed adolescents. Arch Gen Psychiatry 1999;56:573–9.

[24] Young JL, Mufson L, Davies M. Efficacy of interpersonal psychotherapy—adolescent skills training: an indicated preventive intervention for depression. J Child Psychol Psychiatry 2006;47(12):1254–62.

[25] Klerman GL, Weissman MM, Rounsaville BJ, et al. Interpersonal psychotherapy of depression. Northvale (NJ): Jason Aronson, Inc; 1984.

[26] Weissman MM, Markowitz JC, Klerman GL. Comprehensive guide to interpersonal psychotherapy. New York: Basic Books; 2000.

[27] Rosselló J, Bernal G. The efficacy of cognitive-behavioral and interpersonal treatments for depression in Puerto Rican adolescents. J Consult Clin Psychol 1999;67(5):734–45.

[28] Mufson L, Dorta KP, Wickramaratne P, et al. A randomized effectiveness trial of interpersonal psychotherapy for depressed adolescents. Arch Gen Psychiatry 2004;61:577–84.

[29] Wilfley DE, Mackenzie KR, Welch R, et al. Interpersonal psychotherapy for group. New York: Basic Books; 2000.

[30] Stuart S, O'Hara MW, Blehar C. Mental disorders associated with childbearing: report of the biennial meeting of the Marce Society. Psychopharmacol Bull 1998;34:333–8.

[31] Verdeli H, Clougherty KF, Bolton P, et al. Adapting group interpersonal psychotherapy for a developing country: experience in rural Uganda. World Psychiatry 2003;2(2):114–20.

[32] Mufson L, Gallagher T, Dorta KP, et al. A group adaptation of interpersonal psychotherapy for depressed adolescents. Am J Psychother 2004;58(2):220–37.

[33] War Child Holland. 2005. Available at: http://www.warchild.nl. Accessed February 8, 2007.

[34] McCarty CA, Weisz JR. Effects of psychotherapy for depression in children and adolescents: what we can (and can't) learn from meta-analysis and component profiling. J Am Acad Child Adolesc Psychiatry 2007;46(7):879–86.

ELSEVIER
SAUNDERS

Child Adolesc Psychiatric Clin N Am
17 (2008) 625–640

CHILD AND
ADOLESCENT
PSYCHIATRIC CLINICS
OF NORTH AMERICA

Acute Interventions for Refugee Children and Families

Melissa J. Brymer, PhD, PsyD*,
Alan M. Steinberg, PhD, Jo Sornborger, PsyD,
Christopher M. Layne, PhD, Robert S. Pynoos, MD, MPH

*National Center for Child Traumatic Stress, University of California, Los Angeles,
11150 West Olympic Boulevard, Suite 650, Los Angeles, CA 90064, USA*

At the end of 2006, there were 32.9 million refugees, asylum seekers, internally displaced persons, returnees, and stateless people. Of these, approximately 45% were minors under the age of 18 years. Refugees made up nearly one third (9.9 million) of these individuals [1]. Refugee groups in particular tend to have histories of pervasive loss, including home, material belongings, family, friends, neighborhood and school communities, values, daily routines, culture, social status, and opportunities for advancement [2]. Refugee children often have experienced extensive exposure to traumatic events and severe adversities that have taken place in their countries of origin, while fleeing to their host countries, and after arrival in the host country [2]. These three periods have been termed "preflight," "flight," and "resettlement," respectively [3].

Preflight

Refugee children may have been exposed to severe war-related trauma and deprivation, including physical assault, physical injury, persecution, work in forced labor camps, severe malnutrition, severe cold, and lack of access to education, social relationships, and health care. Many also have witnessed horrific events and atrocities, including the execution, torture, physical abuse, rape, humiliation, or arrest of loved ones. Moreover, many have suffered traumatic losses, including forced separations from family members and close friends, the traumatic deaths or disappearances of

---

* Corresponding author.
E-mail address: mbrymer@mednet.ucla.edu (M.J. Brymer).

1056-4993/08/$ - see front matter © 2008 Elsevier Inc. All rights reserved.
doi:10.1016/j.chc.2008.02.007   *childpsych.theclinics.com*

loved ones, the destruction or abandonment of homes and neighborhoods, loss of social status, loss of income and consequent poverty, and the loss of precious belongings, such as beloved pets and toys [4,5].

Subgroups of refugee children have been deployed exploitatively in armed conflicts as combatants, messengers, porters, or cooks or have been forced into marriage or recruited for sexual purposes. Latest estimates indicate that more than 250,000 children under the age of 18 years fall into this category [6]. Child soldiers are at high risk for exposure as direct victims of, witnesses to, or forced perpetrators of severe trauma such as violent death (including mass killings), physical injury, torture, malnutrition and starvation, and rape and associated risk for HIV infection. These experiences place them at risk for posttraumatic stress, anxiety and depressive reactions, substance abuse, and suicidal ideation, as well as for major disruptions in their development, including education, employment, and family and civic life [3].

Flight

Refugee children also are at high risk for exposure to trauma, loss, and severe hardships while in flight, which is characterized by instability and unpredictability. Separation of children from caregivers during or after refugee flight has been linked to a number of adverse outcomes. In particular, unaccompanied minors report significantly higher rates of trauma exposure and associated depression, anxiety, and posttraumatic stress symptoms than do accompanied refugee minors [2].

A study of Palestinian adolescents exposed to political violence found that those who reported living in refugee camps had higher rates of depression than their violence-exposed peers living in cities, towns, and villages [7]. Notably, refugee camps may vary greatly in their levels of organization, sanitation, available resources, and service provision. Traumatic events, including exposure to violence, attempted or completed suicide, separations from family members, and exploitation, may be commonplace [3]. Distress in caregivers may be of particular concern, especially in regard to potential impairments in parental supervision and care-taking. A study of 297 young refugee mothers living in a refugee camp revealed that 36% screened positive for a mental disorder [8].

Resettlement

Newly resettled immigrants experience ongoing separations from loved ones, loss of contact with their native cultures and homelands, and major disruptions in their daily lives. Stress of acculturation involves accommodating to a new language and new foods, cultural and political norms, and religious traditions and practices. Other challenges may include experiencing stigmatization and discrimination, locating available services, learning new customs, and establishing new social relationships. Children's tendency to acquire new languages more rapidly than their parents often places them in the role of "cultural brokers" between adult family members and the host culture by acting as translators and advocates. Differences between generations in language facility and in acculturation may create significant tensions between younger and older generations of immigrants [9]. Newly immigrant children can also be at risk for exposure to community violence in their new neighborhoods.

Interventions with refugee children and their families

Acute psychosocial interventions for refugee children fall on a continuum ranging from services designed to meet the basic needs of an entire population to specialized services for those needing psychiatric care. Current consensus is that community-based psychosocial models are the most efficient and cost effective, adhering to the philosophy that most refugee children and their families will manifest resilience and not need specialized psychiatric services. Community-based programs typically are embedded in existing infrastructures, precluding the establishment of redundant systems [10]. Such programs tend to include community involvement, making these programs more culturally competent.

Efforts to intervene with refugee children have been complicated by at least five major factors [11]:

1. There is a scarcity of rigorously conducted treatment outcome studies with refugee children.
2. It can be difficult to establish appropriate standards of mental health care for this high-risk, underserved population.
3. Practitioners who provide services to refugee populations often lack both basic knowledge about posttraumatic stress disorder (PTSD) and traumatic grief and training in implementing trauma- and grief-focused interventions [12].
4. Refugee children are unlikely to use mental health services because of a variety of barriers.
5. Refugee children experience a wide range of emotional and behavioral problems stemming from exposure to a broad range of stresses and adversities. Problems among refugee children have been found to include anxiety, posttraumatic stress, and depression reactions, recurring nightmares, insomnia, eating disorders, secondary enuresis, externalizing problems, introversion, academic difficulties, and somatic problems.

Studies consistently report significantly higher rates of distress in refugee girls than in refugee boys of the same age [2,7]. Given prevalence estimates of posttraumatic stress reactions ranging between 50% and 90% [3], Birman and colleagues [11] emphasize that many refugee children are in need of trauma-informed treatment and services.

These findings have led clinical researchers to advocate for holistic, comprehensive services that address children's mental health difficulties in their natural environments, including family, school, and other community settings, as well as in social service sectors [9,11,13]. Recommendations for comprehensive services include the incorporation of outreach services and systematic screening for trauma and loss exposure as well as internalizing and externalizing problems. They also include addressing language and other barriers and offering a more extensive array and modalities of mental health services, including community-based psychosocial programs, youth-led peer support and mentoring programs, and outpatient, community, and school-based services. In addition, the literature indicates the need for the adoption of more culturally and developmentally sensitive interventions, increasing access to services [2], implementing interventions that take advantage of naturally occurring community resources [13], and programs that avoid stigmatizing and labeling [3].

Acute interventions for traumatized children

There currently is a critical need for rigorous research on acute interventions for children, adolescents, and families affected by traumatic events [14]. Many of the theoretic perspectives from the general child and adolescent trauma literature and specific principles underlying child and adolescent trauma- and grief-focused interventions have been applied to the design of currently used acute interventions. These interventions can be grouped into several categories.

First, community-based approaches involve working with communities and service systems to deliver psychosocial interventions. These approaches have included psychoeducation, consultation with and training of school personnel, media, and parents, establishment of crisis hotlines, and linkage with available resources [10,15].

Second, art therapies have included the use of drawings of aspects of traumatic experiences, retelling of the child's experiences, discussion of misperceptions, blame, shame, and guilt, and enhancing positive coping strategies. Massage therapy and other expressive therapies (eg, dance, movement, and music) have also been used.

Third, trauma- and grief-focused cognitive behavioral approaches have been employed. These approaches typically have included such strategies as psychoeducation, relaxation, affective modulation, cognitive coping and processing, trauma narrative, various forms of exposure, mastery of trauma reminders, conjoint child-parent sessions, enhancement of future safety and development, and specialized interventions to address traumatic grief reactions [16,17].

Fourth, debriefing strategies have included reconstruction of the event, identification of thoughts and feelings about the event, psychoeducation and normalization, and information on coping [18,19]. During the past decade, research on debriefing techniques has indicated mixed effectiveness [20]. There has been limited empirical support for other approaches and a pressing need for a comprehensive operational guide for conducting acute interventions involving children, adolescents, adults, and families after trauma.

A public mental health approach to mass trauma

Advances in the assessment of traumatized children and adolescents, improved understanding of their posttrauma reactions, and the development and testing of strategies of intervention have set the stage for a modern public mental health approach to child populations affected by mass trauma [21,22]. The first phase of this approach is the conduct of a community-based needs assessment to determine the extent of trauma and loss exposure and to identify different high-risk exposure groups, the degree of current adverse psychosocial difficulties, and the need for and availability of community resources. A useful community-oriented assessment tool is the *Rapid Assessment of Mental Health Needs of Refugees, Displaced and Other Populations Affected by Conflict and Post-Conflict Situations* [23]. Assessments need to be designed to be contextually relevant and appropriate for the local culture through the involvement of local stakeholders in its development. Needs assessments should be performed in conjunction with the provision of psychological first aid (PFA) provided directly to children and their families [24,25]. Periodic screenings (surveillance) permit ongoing identification of affected children or groups at risk and provide a mechanism for monitoring the course of recovery and the type and quality of services used.

The initial screening should include basic information about exposure to trauma and loss; health and safety needs; specific questions about high-risk experiences (eg, direct threats to life; being trapped or injured; witnessing grotesque injury or death; being separated from family members or caregivers); cultural, religious, political, and socioeconomic issues; current adversities; and current behavioral and functional difficulties (eg, impaired daily functioning). In addition to providing useful triage information, screening, within the framework of PFA, serves a psychoeducational function. Sharing of aggregate information derived from data collected by governmental and other public health agencies can help promote more judicious allocation of resources and support for intervention efforts [22].

The public mental health approach to intervention includes three tiers. Tier 1 provides PFA to the affected child and community population. Such support may include stabilizing the child, family, or community milieu; addressing immediate health, mental health and safety concerns; providing practical assistance; enhancing coping strategies and the use of community and social support resources; providing information on common stress reactions and cautions about risk-related behavior; and linkage with available support resources. Tier 2 provides more specialized support and treatment for those who have moderate-to-severe persisting distress and associated impairment. Tier 2 includes five focal areas of intervention: traumatic experiences; trauma and loss reminders; traumatic bereavement; current stresses and adversities; and assistance in maintaining normal developmental progression. Tier 3 provides specialized psychiatric services for youth who require immediate and/or intensive treatment [26].

These three tiers of intervention are designed to complement one another and, where appropriate, to link together to provide continuity of care. For example, Tier 1 interventions can educate the school community regarding signs of trauma and loss-related distress and can provide information regarding referrals to qualified school and community professionals. Tier 2 and Tier 3 activities can benefit mutually from active linkages between school and community mental health professionals. For example, a psychiatrist can prescribe antidepressant medication and consult with school counselors regarding depressed students.

The development of Psychological First Aid

In response to the need for more structured acute intervention guidelines, the National Child Traumatic Stress Network and the National Center for Posttraumatic Stress Disorder have developed the *Psychological First Aid (PFA) Field Operations Guide*, second edition [27], an acute intervention that is supportive, nonintrusive, and strongly problem- and solution-focused. PFA is an evidence-informed modular approach for assisting children, adolescents, and families in reducing the initial distress caused by catastrophic events and fostering short- and long-term adaptive functioning. It is derived from a developmental model of child traumatic stress [28,29] and relies on a number of basic principles that have received broad empirical support for facilitating positive adaptation following stress: (1) promoting safety; (2) promoting calming; (3) promoting self- and community efficacy; (4) promoting connectedness; and (5) instilling hope [30].

Promoting safety

Physiological and psychological responses to trauma and trauma reminders trigger fears of recurrence, feelings of helplessness, and concerns over safety. Traumatic events also interfere with young children's sense of a "protective shield" [25]. When children feel unsafe, they can regress to earlier developmental behaviors and experience separation anxiety and disruptions of attachment with primary caregivers. PFA strategies are intended to help children with practical safety issues and to restore a sense of safety by helping them manage and reduce these physiological and psychological responses, enhance parent/caregiver capacity for protecting and supporting their children, re-establish a family routine to increase predictability, and reduce exposure to further trauma and reminders.

Promoting calming

Traumatic events and losses create anxiety and emotional arousal that can interfere with sleep, decision making, attention and concentration, mood, and effective coping. For children who are having difficulty calming down, anxiety management techniques (eg, breathing, muscle relaxation, cognitive restructuring) and problem-solving strategies can be useful. Additionally, establishing routines, assisting parents in their roles, and encouraging normal child activities can help appreciably in promoting a sense of calm for children.

Promoting self- and community efficacy

Disaster research has indicated that loss of personal, social, and economic resources is associated with diminished perception of self-efficacy and confidence in the community's ability to promote recovery [31,32]. To address issues of self-efficacy, PFA strategies include providing practical assistance, encouraging constructive activities and positive coping, assisting in problem-solving, promoting proactive engagement in community activities, providing assistance in receiving and giving social support, and linking with community services.

Promoting connectedness

The objective of connecting individuals and families with community supports is based on research indicating that social support is related to improved emotional well-being and recovery following trauma [33,34]. Promoting family and community connectedness has many benefits, including increasing different types of social support (eg, emotional closeness, physical assistance, and material support) and expanding the range of community networks and enhancing family cohesion [17]. PFA strategies are directed toward keeping individuals connected to their family and community and identifying and assisting those who may be displaced, separated, or lack adequate support. Specific strategies are recommended to enhance family connectedness through mutual understanding and acceptance of differences in family members' exposure and course of recovery.

Instilling hope

Instilling hope has been identified as a crucial component of postdisaster recovery, because those who maintain optimism, positive expectancy, and a feeling of confidence that life and self are predictable are likely to have more favorable outcomes after experiencing mass trauma [35]. Many of the PFA intervention strategies are designed to promote a sense of hopefulness about the future and expectations of recovery. These strategies include connecting children and families with services to rebuild their lives and encouraging proactive problem-solving and prosocial community activities. Providing information about expectable reactions and strategies to manage them also can contribute to hopefulness for the future.

Psychological First Aid

The basic principles, objectives, and techniques of PFA were designed to meet four basic standards. These are:

1. Consistent with research evidence on risk and resilience following trauma
2. Applicable and practical in field settings
3. Appropriate for developmental levels across the lifespan
4. Culturally informed and deliverable in a flexible manner

PFA is intended for use by disaster response workers who provide assistance under the auspices of a variety of disaster relief agencies and organizations. It is designed to be appropriate for use in diverse settings, including refugee camps, family assistance centers, schools, hospitals, homes, and faith-based and other community settings (eg, youth centers, child play areas).

PFA or other acute interventions should be imbedded in a system of care to ensure that providers coordinate with other governmental and nongovernmental organizations that are providing services for children and families. This provision also promotes provider coordination with lead agencies and compliance with guidelines or incident command procedures. Programs should be integrated into existing structures to avoid parallel systems or stand-alone programs. Training in PFA or other acute interventions should be conducted before services are delivered, and a mechanism for follow-up should be in place to make sure interventions are being implemented and adapted appropriately for the population served. PFA providers should work with cultural and community leaders to understand the cultural norms and sociopolitical history of the area and to adapt PFA interventions accordingly [36].

The core actions of PFA include:

1. Contact and engagement
2. Safety and comfort
3. Stabilization
4. Information gathering
5. Practical assistance
6. Connection with social supports
7. Information on coping
8. Linkage with collaborative services

The core action of *Contact and Engagement* includes responding to and initiating contacts in a nonintrusive, compassionate, and helpful manner, maintaining a calm presence, and maximizing the participation of members of affected communities. Providers need to identify those groups who have had to live with continual social stigmas in their communities (eg, people at risk for human rights violations, survivors who have experienced gender discrimination, ethnic or linguistic minorities, people in institutions, and those who have disabilities) and be wary of heightening those stigmas [36].

The core action of *Safety and Comfort* includes enhancing survivors' immediate and ongoing safety by helping provide both physical and emotional comfort. This component includes providing and clarifying risk-related information, and information about the current disaster response and available services. PFA providers should identify current circumstances that may affect a child's safety (eg, current human rights violations, potential threat of landmines, lack of access to basic needs or health care) and coordinate with organizations that can help address such issues [36]. When working with refugee children, PFA providers may have to work with other professionals to make sure that the environment in which the children are living is safe and that basic routines are provided for children. This action may include recommending that safe play areas be developed, ensuring that education is offered to all children, and facilitating family routines and tasks. In working with refugee children, attending to family reunification and adhering to guidelines for unaccompanied minors is the most important priority to ensure these children's safety. Helping survivors identify various trauma reminders and reducing unnecessary exposure to additional reminders also can help promote their sense of safety.

Sexual and gender-based violence is recognized as a pervasive problem worldwide and is more pronounced in situations of war, political conflicts, and in refugee/displacement settings. PFA providers need to handle these situations with great sensitivity and be aware of potential security issues for community members and for themselves [37]. In particular, provider organizations should conduct a situation analysis of how the community and government perceives and responds to survivors of sexual and gender-based violence and to evaluate whether the current physical layout of the settlement increases the risk for women and children. Providers need to ensure additional safeguards to protect the safety and confidentiality of women and children who have been targets of such abuse. This activity may include linking these survivors with others in the community who are advocates for protecting them from additional harm or stigma.

Worry about the safety of loved ones and concern about protecting them from harm is common after mass trauma. Survivors may be confronted with the death or serious injuries of loved ones, or with missing loved ones, and PFA offers strategies and techniques to assist survivors through such processes as reporting or searching for missing loved ones, receiving death notification, and participating in body identification.

To address a survivor's emotional comfort, a PFA provider may have to address issues of acute grief reactions and traumatic grief. When addressing grief issues, providers need to facilitate appropriate communal, cultural, spiritual, and specific religious practices. PFA providers typically get questions from parents or community leaders about how to talk to children about death and about children's attendance at funerals, memorials, or gravesites. When providers are working with grieving survivors, it is important that they have an appreciation of the mourning rituals and practices of the community before conducting any specific interventions. It also is important for providers to understand what community leaders have been communicating to children and to help clarify any misinformation that has been given. As Yule [38] noted, PFA providers may help educate the community about children's understanding of death and that giving them misinformation (eg, their parents went abroad to work) would be harmful to the child's recovery. The *Psychological First Aid (PFA) Field Operations Guide* provides strategies for parents/caregivers in talking with their children about death and in assisting their children with feelings of loss.

The core action of *Stabilization* is to calm and orient emotionally overwhelmed and distraught survivors. Although it is not assumed that most individuals affected by traumatic events will require stabilization, PSA offers grounding techniques to focus individuals on the present and to reduce distress. The goal of these intervention strategies is to reduce the immediate extreme distress and facilitate decision making and the performance of important current activities.

An important feature of PFA is the use of *Information-Gathering* strategies throughout the intervention that allow the provider to tailor and address the intervention to the specific needs and concerns of affected children and families. Some of the categories include separation from loved ones; death or injury of loved ones; safety concerns, health and mental health; availability of social and community supports; and sleep problems. The *Psychological First Aid (PFA) Field Operations Guide* includes specific courses of action to be pursued in relation to information obtained. PFA providers are cautioned against asking for in-depth descriptions of traumatic experiences.

The core action of *Practical Assistance* aims to offer practical help to survivors in addressing immediate needs and concerns. To achieve this goal, problem-solving strategies are used to identify the survivor's most immediate needs or problems, clarify these needs, discuss an action plan, and provide assistance in acting to address the needs. Providing survivors with needed resources can increase a sense of empowerment, hope, and restored dignity. Assisting children and families with practical needs is a central component of PFA.

The goal of *Connection with Social Supports* is to facilitate and mobilize natural support systems to bring individuals together. This component includes facilitating and empowering existing community structures and organizations (eg, local traditional healers, religious institutions, schools, women's grass-root organizations) and connecting survivors to these networks that promote well-being and recovery [10]. PFA providers may help facilitate formal or informal groups to help survivors meet their collective needs and to foster natural coping. This facilitation also ensures that coping is appropriate to the cultural values of the community and can be continued after the acute phase ends. For adolescents, being empowered to lead groups and to implement prosocial activities in their communities has been shown to help provide a sense of meaning and purpose and to accelerate recovery [39].

PFA strategies are directed at identifying disruptions of social networks and decreasing social isolation by identifying and educating those who lack strong support and who are likely to be more socially isolated. PFA strategies may help marginalized groups be more integrated or included in community networks. For refugee children, helping them with a sense of belonging and connection to their new school is especially important [40].

The goal of information on coping is to provide psychoeducation about stress reactions and coping to reduce distress and promote adaptive functioning. Simple relaxation techniques can be taught and used in acute-care settings. An important part of this core action includes sharing information with families about the need to establish routines to the extent possible and the importance for family members to be understanding and tolerant of differences in their reactions. Other intervention strategies include helping with developmental disruptions, anger management, highly negative emotions (guilt and shame), sleep problems, and problems with substance use. Promoting the use of effective coping strategies includes integrating local traditional practices when appropriate.

Linkage with Collaborative Services includes immediate referral for serious health and mental health issues, referral to community resources (eg, childcare, youth centers, remedial educational programs, job training, local traditional healers, religious and spiritual institutions, legal services, social services), and strategies for the promotion of continuity in helping relationships. PFA providers should make sure that the child and family understand the purpose for the referral and that the services are available.

The Psychological First Aid (PFA) Field Operations Guide includes a number of handouts that provide information for children, adolescents, adults, and parents/caregivers about common reactions after disasters, seeking and giving support, positive and negative coping strategies, tips for assisting children at the infant/toddler, preschool, school-age, and adolescent levels, basic relaxation techniques, substance use and abuse, and self-care strategies for providers implementing PFA. These materials provide important information that survivors can use over the weeks and months of recovery. PFA providers should ensure that the handouts are culturally appropriate and make recommendations to their organizations about any needed adaptations. Where multiple languages are spoken, the handouts should be translated to meet the needs of all linguistic groups.

The *Psychological First Aid (PFA) Field Operations Guide*, adaptations for different service systems (eg, community religious professionals, school personel), translations, accompanying training materials, and evaluation tools are available at www.NCTSN.org. Materials and resources related to refugee children and families also are available on this Website.

Skills for Psychological Recovery

The National Child Traumatic Stress Network and the National Center for PTSD currently are developing a second field operations guide for the intermediate stage of disaster response, *Skills for Psychological Recovery* (SPR). This guide is being developed to meet criteria for the Federal Emergency Management Agency/Substance Abuse and Mental Health Services Administration Crisis Counseling Programs that are funded after a federally declared disaster in the United States. This intervention is for use from 2 months to more than 1 year postdisaster and is an example of a Tier 2 intervention. SPR includes several core, empirically-based skill sets that have been shown to help with a variety of postdisaster issues. Research suggests that a skills-building approach is more effective than supportive counseling, and consequently SPR embodies problem- and solution-focused approaches. The core actions included in SPR are:

- *Information gathering:* a method to gather information to determine the need for referral, to identify and prioritize current needs, problems, and concerns, and to select and implement an appropriate SPR intervention
- *Building problem-solving skills:* a four-step method to clarify a problem, identify a number of ways to solve it, and a way to choose and try a solution that is likely to be helpful in addressing the problem
- *Promoting helpful thinking:* a technique to identify upsetting thoughts and ways to replace these thoughts with less upsetting ones
- *Promoting positive activities:* a strategy to identify and engage in positive, constructive, and pleasurable activities
- *Building and maintaining healthy connections:* a strategy to identify and engage people who can help in feeling understood and supported in dealing with problems, and ways to help others
- *Managing distressing reactions:* ways to manage and reduce distressing physical and emotional reactions to upsetting situations, such as reactions to trauma and loss reminders and to ongoing stress and adversity
- *Linking with available services:* a way to link with services that can help address current pressing needs and practical concerns

Each core action includes a number of provider skill steps that comprise the core action. For example, the information gathering section includes the following skill steps:

1. Explain the rationale for information gathering.
2. Use the SPR screening form to gather information and prioritize the survivor's current needs, problems, and concerns.
3. Summarize the information gathered.
4. Make urgently needed referrals or referral for available services.
5. Work with the survivor to plan and implement an SPR intervention for a prioritized problem.

SPR interventions are intended for use with children, adolescents, parents/caregivers, families, and adults exposed to mass trauma. SPR also can be provided to first responders and other disaster-relief workers. It is designed for use by mental health and other disaster-response workers who provide assistance as part of an organized disaster-response effort. These providers may be embedded in a variety of settings, including crisis counseling programs, community mental health, primary and emergency health care, school mental health programs, faith-based organizations, community recovery programs, and governmental and nongovernmental programs and services. As with PFA, SPR includes a set of appendices on delivery in a group modality and a variety of handouts to be used in helping survivors gain the core skills. Progressive development of these interventions is based on a staged approach to providing increasingly extended and in-depth interventions over the course of posttrauma adaptation and recovery and on the recognition that most survivors will not need extensive mental health treatment.

Future directions

Establishing the evidence base for PFA and SPR will need to be done in progressive stages that correspond to a number of basic research questions. These questions address issues ranging from the evaluation of training to assessment of the short- and long-term benefits for survivors and on the overall system and community disaster response efforts. Among the overarching research questions are the following:

1. What types of training methods and resources are needed to disseminate these interventions effectively?
2. Do trained providers implement these interventions with fidelity?
3. Can these interventions be delivered effectively and received by survivors in disaster settings, including refugee camps?
4. Does implementing the intervention with fidelity assist in realizing each of the specific intervention objectives (internal evaluation)?
5. Does implementing the intervention lead to improved outcomes as compared with other intervention practices (external evaluation)?
6. Does implementing the intervention in a postdisaster setting improve the overall effectiveness and efficiency of the disaster response efforts in that setting?

Addressing these research questions will require the use of a variety of research strategies and metrics, including the use of focus groups; evaluation of the transference of knowledge, skills, and attitudes using a variety of training platforms; prospective longitudinal designs and randomized, controlled studies to evaluate the potential benefits of the intervention; and formal program evaluation to examine system and community outcomes.

Attention should be directed toward identifying and assessing intervention components that may benefit survivors after the intervention has ended. These components include (1) linkage with collaborative services, (2) use of handouts by survivors over time, and (3) ongoing use by survivors of knowledge and skills acquired during the intervention.

The authors currently are developing PFA provider and survivor evaluation forms to gather information from providers on problem areas addressed and components used in delivering PFA and from survivors in regard to the perceived helpfulness of the contact, what components of the assistance were seen to be most helpful, whether there were parts of the assistance that were not helpful or were perceived as harmful, and whether some types of assistance were desired but not received. Given the pressing needs of refugee children and their families, it is imperative to establish an evidence-base for acute interventions. PFA is a promising practice that recently has gained national and international support, but studies now are needed to establish its effectiveness.

References

[1] United Nations High Commissioner for Refugees. 2006 global trends: refugees, asylum-seekers, returnees, internally displaced and stateless persons. Available at: http://www.unhcr.org/statistics/STATISTICS/4676a71d4.pdf. 2007. Accessed January 13, 2008.
[2] Derlyun I, Broekaert E. Different perspectives on emotional and behavioural problems in unaccompanied refugee children and adolescents. Ethn Health 2007;12(2):141–62.
[3] Lustig SL, Kia-Keating M, Grant Knight W, et al. Review of child and adolescent refugee mental health. J Am Acad Child Adolesc Psychiatry 2004;1:24–36.
[4] Sack WH, Him C, Dickason D. Twelve-year follow-up study of Khmer youths who suffered massive war trauma as children. J Am Acad Child Adolesc Psychiatry 1999;38(9):1173–9.
[5] Weine S, Becker DF, McGlashan TH, et al. Adolescent survivors of "ethnic cleansing": observations on the first year in America. J Am Acad Child Adolesc Psychiatry 1995;34(9):1153–9.
[6] UNICEF. Adult wars, child soldiers: voices of children involved in armed conflict in the East Asia and Pacific Region. Thailand: United Nations Children's Fund; 2002. p. 6.
[7] Giacaman R, Shannon HS, Saab H, et al. Individual and collective exposure to political violence: Palestinian adolescents coping with conflict. Eur J Public Health 2007;17(4):361–8.
[8] Rahman A, Hafeez A. Suicidal feelings run high among mothers in refugee camps: a cross-sectional survey. Acta Psychiatr Scand 2003;108(5):392–3.
[9] Hodes M. Psychologically distressed refugee children in the United Kingdom. Child Psychology & Psychiatry Review 2000;5(2):57–68.
[10] Kos AM. Activating community resources for the well being of children and stability. In: Friedman MJ, Kos AM, editors. Promoting the psychosocial well-being of children following war and terrorism. The Netherlands: IOS Press; 2005. p. 121–61.
[11] Birman D, Ho J, Pulley E, et al. Mental health interventions for refugee children in resettlement white paper II (2005). National Child Traumatic Stress Network Refugee Trauma Task Force, 2005. Available at: www.NCTSN.org. Accessed December 15, 2007.
[12] Weine SM, Henderson SW. Rethinking the role of posttraumatic stress disorder in refugee mental health services. In: Corales TA, editor. Trends in posttraumatic stress disorder research. Hauppauge (NY): Nova Science Publishers; 2005. p. 157–83.

[13] Ethntholt KA, Yule W. Practitioner review: assessment and treatment of refugee children and adolescents who have experienced war-related trauma. J Child Psychol Psychiatry 2006;47(12):1197–210.

[14] Steinberg AM, Brymer MJ, Steinberg JR, et al. Conducting research on children and adolescents after mass trauma. In: Norris F, Friedman M, Galea S, et al, editors. Methods for disaster mental health research. New York: Guildford Press; 2006. p. 243–53.

[15] Macy RD, Behar L, Paulson R, et al. Community-based, acute posttraumatic stress management: a description and evaluation of a psychosocial-intervention continuum. Harv Rev Psychiatry 2004;12:217–28.

[16] Cohen JA, Mannarino AP, Deblinger E. Treating trauma and traumatic grief in children and adolescents. New York: Guildford Press; 2006.

[17] Layne CM, Pynoos RS, Saltzman WR, et al. Trauma/grief-focused group psychotherapy: school-based postwar intervention with traumatized Bosnian adolescents. Group Dynamics: Theory, Research and Practice 2001;5:277–90.

[18] Morgan KE, White PR. The functions of art-making in CISD with children and youth. Int J Emerg Ment Health 2003;5:61–76.

[19] Stallard P, Velleman R, Salter E, et al. A randomised controlled trial to determine the effectiveness of an early psychological intervention with children involved in road traffic accidents. J Child Psychol Psychiatry 2006;47:127–34.

[20] McNally RJ, Bryant RA, Ehlers A. Does early psychological intervention promote recovery from posttraumatic stress? Psychological Science in the Public Interest 2003;4:45–79.

[21] Pynoos RS, Goenjian AK, Steinberg AM. Strategies of disaster intervention for children and adolescents. In: Hobfoll SE, deVries MW, editors. Extreme stress and communities: impact and prevention. Dordrecht (The Netherlands): Kluwer Academic Publishers; 1995. p. 445–71.

[22] Pynoos RS, Goenjian AK, Steinberg AM. A public mental health approach to the post-disaster treatment of children and adolescents. Psychiatr Clin North Am 1998;7:195–210.

[23] Jacobs GA, Revel JP, Reyes G, et al. Development of the rapid assessment of mental health: an international collaboration. In: Reyes G, Jacobs GA, editors. Refugee mental health. Handbook of international disaster psychology, vol. 3. Westport (CT): Praeger Publishers; 2006. p. 129–40.

[24] Pynoos RS, Nadar K. Psychological first aid & treatment approach to children exposed to community violence: research implications. J Trauma Stress 1988;1(4):445–73.

[25] Pynoos RS, Steinberg AM, Brymer MJ. Children and disasters: public mental health approaches. In: Ursano RJ, Fullerton CS, Weisaeth L, et al, editors. Textbook of disaster psychiatry. Cambridge (UK): Cambridge University Press; 2007. p. 48–68.

[26] Saltzman WR, Layne CM, Steinberg AS, et al. Developing a culturally and ecologically sound intervention program for youth exposed to war and terrorism. Child Adolesc Psychiatr Clin N Am 2003;12:319–42.

[27] Brymer MJ, Jacobs A, Layne C, et al. Psychological first aid: field operations guide. 2nd edition. National Child Traumatic Stress Network & National Center for PTSD; 2006. Available at: www.nctsn.org, and www.ncptsd.va.gov.

[28] Pynoos RS, Steinberg AM, Wraith R. A developmental model of childhood traumatic stress. In: Cicchetti D, Cohen DJ, editors. Manual of developmental psychopathology. New York: John Wiley & Sons; 1995. p. 72–93.

[29] Pynoos RS, Steinberg AM, Piacentini JC. Developmental psychopathology of childhood traumatic stress and implications for associated anxiety disorders. Biol Psychiatry 1999; 46:1542–54.

[30] Hobfoll SE, Watson PE, Ruzek JI, et al. Five essential elements of immediate and mid-term mass trauma intervention: empirical evidence. Psychiatry: Interpersonal and Biological Processes 2007;70:283–315.

[31] Galea S, Ahern J, Resnick H, et al. Psychological sequelae of the September 11 terrorist attacks in New York City. N Engl J Med 2002;346:982–7.

[32] Norris FH, Kaniasty K. Received and perceived social support in times of stress: a test of the social support deterioration deterrence model. J Pers Soc Psychol 1996;71:498–511.

[33] Bleich A, Gelkopf M, Solomon Z. Exposure to terrorism, stress-related mental health symptoms, and coping behaviors among a nationally representative sample in Israel. JAMA 2003;290(5):612–20.

[34] Stein BD, Elliott MN, Jaycox LH, et al. A national longitudinal study of the psychological consequences of the September 11, 2001 terrorist attacks: reactions, impairment, and help-seeking. Psychiatry 2004;67:105–17.

[35] Carver CS. Resilience and thriving: issues, models and linkages. J Soc Issues 1998;54:245–66.

[36] Inter-Agency Standing Committee (IASC). IASC guidelines on mental health and psychosocial support in emergency settings. Geneva (Switzerland): Inter-Agency Standing Committee; 2007.

[37] Reis C, Vann B. Sexual violence against women and children in the context of armed conflict. In: Reyes G, Jacobs GA, editors. Interventions with special needs populations. Handbook of international disaster psychology, vol. 4. Westport (CT): Praeger Publishers; 2006. p. 19–44.

[38] Yule W. Theory, training, and timing: psychosocial interventions in complex emergencies. Int Rev Psychiatry 2006;18(3):259–64.

[39] Pynoos RS, Steinberg AM. Recovery of children and adolescents after exposure to violence: a developmental ecological framework. In: Liberman AF, DeMartino AF, editors. Johnson & Johnson Pediatric Roundtable Series, vol. 6. Interventions for children exposed to violence. New Brunswick (NJ): Johnson & Johnson Pediatric Institute, LLC; 2006. p. 17–43.

[40] Kia-Keating M, Ellis BH. Belonging and connection to school in resettlement: youth refugees, school belonging, and psychosocial adjustment. Clin Child Psychol Psychiatry 2007;12(1):29–43.

ELSEVIER
SAUNDERS

Child Adolesc Psychiatric Clin N Am
17 (2008) 641–664

CHILD AND
ADOLESCENT
PSYCHIATRIC CLINICS
OF NORTH AMERICA

Narrative Exposure Therapy for the Treatment of Traumatized Children and Adolescents (KidNET): From Neurocognitive Theory to Field Intervention

Frank Neuner, PhD*, Claudia Catani, PhD,
Martina Ruf, MA, Elisabeth Schauer, PhD,
Maggie Schauer, PhD, Thomas Elbert, PhD

Department of Psychology, University of Konstanz, Box D25, D-78457 Konstanz, Germany

Current evidence and practice

Violence against children, including maltreatment at home, sexual abuse, and child labor, are common phenomena worldwide. In addition, many children are affected by violence caused by political conflicts, unrest, and war. Current wars are characterized by high levels of deliberate and systematic violence against the civilian population [1], including victimization of women and children. More than 30 countries are affected by current wars, and the populations of many now peaceful countries suffer from the aftermaths of a recent armed conflict. In addition, the number and intensity of environmental disasters is increasing. Environmental disasters mainly affect low-income countries with poor facilities for an adequate emergency response [2]. In some regions, war and environmental disaster co-occur [3], causing severe acute emergencies and a long-lasting mental health impairment in the population.

Although children can be astonishingly resilient even in face of severe disasters and atrocities, high levels of traumatic events increase the risk of developmental difficulties and psychologic disorders. Many studies have shown increased rates of mental disorders in children affected by war [4].

This work was supported by the Ministry of Science, Research and the Arts of Baden-Württemberg, the Deutsche Forschungsgemeinschaft, and the European Refugee Fund.

* Corresponding author.

E-mail address: frank.neuner@uni-konstanz.de (F. Neuner).

doi:10.1016/j.chc.2008.03.001

childpsych.theclinics.com

The most prevalent disorder is posttraumatic stress disorder (PTSD), which consists predominantly of intrusive thoughts, flashbacks, nightmares, avoidance behavior, and increased levels of arousal. The prevalence of PTSD in children in war-affected populations ranges from 20% among Lebanese children who were exposed to bombings and terror attacks [5] to 44% in surviving orphans 10 years after the Rwandan genocide [6]. A survey in the war-affected northeastern region of Sri Lanka showed that 19% to 25% of the Tamil children already were suffering from PTSD before the region was hit by the devastating tsunami flood wave in 2004 [7]. After the tsunami, PTSD rates of 40% were found in communities affected by both war and disaster [8]. In addition, Catani and co-workers [3] found a high level of family violence in these communities. Confirming a general dose–effect model [9], PTSD in children was predicted mainly by the cumulative exposure to trauma including war, disaster, and family violence in this population.

Longitudinal studies show that trauma symptoms in children are more than simply a behavioral problem that dissipates over time as the child matures. Rates of spontaneous remission in traumatized children are remarkably low [10]. In a large proportion of severely war-traumatized children, PTSD can persist for more than 10 years even when the children are living in a safe environment [11]. As a consequence, intervention strategies for severely traumatized children in war-affected populations are necessary to prevent a downward spiral in development. Intervention research in this area is still in its infancy, however, and common practice rarely is informed by scientific knowledge. Even though regions in crisis and refugee camps often attract humanitarian workers from many different countries, psychosocial activities are restricted mostly to interventions such as creative play therapy, the indiscriminate distribution of psychoeducational material, and supportive counseling. Most often, the interventions provided by humanitarian workers and health professionals have been developed ad hoc without a solid theoretic background, and the efficacy of these methods, including play activities, is doubtful [12].

In recent years, knowledge about the treatment of PTSD in children living in high-resource countries has increased rapidly. There now is considerable evidence supporting different variants of cognitive behavioral therapy (CBT) for the treatment of school children who have PTSD resulting from multiple traumatic events, including sexual abuse [13] and other forms of violence [14]. In general, CBT programs include psychoeducation, cognitive interventions, training of affective coping skills, and exposure therapy. Several randomized trials have shown that in treating PTSD symptoms CBT is more effective than standard care, unspecific therapy, or no treatment [15]. Follow-up studies have demonstrated that treatment gains are maintained for up to 2 years [16].

Unfortunately, no randomized controlled study has included child war victims or traumatized refugees. Some pragmatic treatment programs have been developed for use in crises in low-resource countries or in refugee communities. For example the "Children and War: Teaching Recovery Techniques" approach [17] was developed as a trauma-focused group intervention for the context of disaster, war, and refugee populations and was tested in several uncontrolled and nonrandomized controlled studies. In general, trauma-focused group programs showed promising effects with significant reductions of PTSD symptoms [18]. Although clinically significant treatment effects could be demonstrated for disaster victims in uncontrolled studies [19,20] and even in a randomized trial [21], treatment gains were modest and did not seem to be stable over time when applied to refugee children in the United Kingdom [22], and no significant effect was found for refugee children in Gaza [23].

The authors have developed narrative exposure therapy (NET) as a pragmatic, short-term intervention for traumatized victims of war and torture. NET is an individual-level, trauma-focused treatment that, on the one hand, builds on the tradition of testimony therapy developed by Lira and Weinstein to treat the victims of the Pinochet regime in Chile [24]. The key aspect of testimony therapy is the detailed documentation of human rights violations experienced by the survivor of political violence and the use of this testimony for political purposes. On the other hand, NET builds on the principles of current neurocognitive theories of PTSD and cognitive behavioral therapy by adapting the classical form of exposure therapy to meet the needs of traumatized survivors of war and torture. In exposure therapy for PTSD [25], the patient is asked to talk repeatedly about the worst traumatic event in detail while re-experiencing all emotions associated with the event. In the process, most patients undergo habituation of the emotional response to the traumatic memory. This habituation consequently leads to a remission of PTSD symptoms. Typically, victims of organized violence have experienced multiple traumatic events; the authors encountered a child who had seen her brother die from shrapnel wounds and who later was raped. As outlined later in this article, multiple traumatic events can cause a substantial distortion in autobiographic memory with an excessive emotional representation that includes an unsorted batch of stimuli from different memories. It therefore is difficult to differentiate different episodes or to identify a single worst event before treatment. Consequently, in NET, the patient constructs a narration of his or her whole life from early childhood to the present date while focusing on the detailed report of traumatic experiences [26].

Theoretical background: neurocognitive memory theory

The most prominent neurobiologic and cognitive theories of PTSD explain the development of PTSD on the basis of a pathologic distortion of the memory representations of the traumatic event [27–30]. According to Tulving [31], there is a specific store of memories about past events called "episodic memory." Episodic memory involves happenings in particular places at particular times and covers context information about "what," "where," and "when." A unique feature that distinguishes episodic memory from other memory systems is the possibility of consciously re-experiencing previous events in the form of recollective experiences. Most theories of episodic memory separate at least two different bases of episodic knowledge: nondeclarative memory and declarative memory (for a different view see [32]). These memory systems differ in the retrieval of information: declarative (explicit) memory can be retrieved deliberately and accessed verbally, whereas nondeclarative (implicit) memory is activated automatically by environmental or internal cues and affects a person's behavior and experience [33]. Therefore one must distinguish between a declarative episodic memory system (later called "autobiographical representation") and a nondeclarative episodic memory system (later called "sensory-perceptual representation"). In addition, there is good reason to assume that a supervisory structure controls the activity of the memory representations.

Autobiographical representation

The declarative part of episodic memory has been called "autobiographical memory" [34]; other authors have used the terms "verbally accessible memory" [35] or "cold memory" [36]. Autobiographical memory is a highly developed and structured memory system that allows the abundant knowledge about past events to be filed in a highly efficient way. Autobiographical memory is the principal resource for the retrieval of information about one's life and is the main base for the narration of events and life periods. To allow a rapid and organized access of information, this memory is structured in a hierarchical way. At the top of the organization are the lifetime periods that have identifiable beginnings and endings. They represent general knowledge of important other persons, locations, actions, activities, plans, and goals. An example of a lifetime period is "when I was living with Maria" or "when I was working at the farm." One level below the lifetime periods is the memory for general events. General events can be divided into repeated events (eg, "having lunch at the canteen") and specific events (eg, "my first day in school"). These knowledge bases organize the chronologic sequence of single events.

The neurobiologic correlate of autobiographical memory cannot be identified as a single brain structure. Rather, long-term storage of autobiographic and other declarative knowledge depends on widespread neocortical neuronal activity. This complex neuronal network underlies a special organization including specific rules and consistencies. This organization allows the effective storage of the vast amount of knowledge a human being can acquire. At the same time, this complex organization makes this network slow to integrate new incoming information, especially new events that are incompatible with previous knowledge.

The key brain structure related to autobiographic memories is the hippo-campus. The hippocampus itself is not the permanent store of declarative memory, but it has a central function in the consolidation of memory within the first 4 weeks of the event. In this period, the information is located to a wide neocortical network [37]. Several neuroscientists assume that the function of the hippocampus is to construct a meaningful episodic represen-tation of the dynamics of the situation in a spatiotemporal context [38]. McClelland and coworkers [39] suggested that the hippocampus is especially important for the coding of information that contradicts previously learned knowledge. They assume that the neocortical system is slow to integrate contradictory information, because that information undermines strict rules and consistencies. In this context, the hippocampus may permit the forma-tion of a rapid representation of the event and gradually expose the neocortical system to the new information. In this way the network can be reorganized slowly to integrate the new information.

Sensory-perceptual representation

When a person thinks about a past life event, it is be possible that he or she both retrieves abstract knowledge about what has happened and also can imagine the event in the form of a recollective experience [31]. Thus, in addition to declarative autobiographic facts, people can access directly the sensory and emotional information about past events stored in their minds, including an awareness of the subjective time when the event hap-pened. The retrieval of this sensory information is fundamentally different from the retrieval of autobiographic information. Whereas the contextual facts stored in autobiographic memory are retrieved as verbally accessible knowledge, the retrieval of sensory information is perceived as an experience of the information itself. For example, a person who has a vivid memory of his first day at a beach actually might see the water in front of his eyes and re-experience the excitement of that moment when thinking back on the event. This type of information is provided by a sensory-perceptual repre-sentation of the event (other authors have used such terms as "hot memory" [36], "situationally accessible memory," [35] or "event-specific knowledge" [34]). The sensory-perceptual representation itself does not contain any context information about single events, but a close tie to the corresponding autobiographical representations offers a spatial and temporal context for this memory. As a consequence, the activation of the sensory-perceptual details of an event usually is accompanied by the activation of autobio-graphical knowledge about the sequence of the event and the location of the event in lifetime periods.

Obviously, a vivid and detailed recollection is not possible for all events experienced in a life. For everyday events that have a minor meaning for the person involved, the sensory-perceptual representations usually only last minutes or hours [40]. The enduring storage of sensory-perceptual representations happens only for events stored in a highly emotional state, because they are significant for the achievement or failure of a person's individual goals [34].

Lang's [41] bio-informational theory of emotions offers a good framework for understanding the nature of sensory-perceptual representations and their relationship to emotions. In this view, emotions are represented mentally as associative networks. These representations consist of sensory information about the stimuli present in the past situation in different modalities (eg, visual, auditory, olfactory). At the same time, this network contains information about the cognitive and affective evaluation of the stimuli and the corresponding physiologic responses. Fig. 1 provides a sensory-perceptual representation of a person's memory of a special moment on a beach. The items of these networks are connected so that the activation of single items causes the spreading activation of connected items. Items of the representation can be activated either by external stimuli that share features of the memory (eg, being at the sea again) or by thinking deeply about the event. A recollective experience of the memory can follow, because single sensory elements are interconnected and therefore are likely to be activated together. In addition, the recollective experience can be accompanied by the vivid sensation of the emotions, cognitions, and physiologic responses represented in the memory, because they are associated with the sensory elements. While remembering that day, the person actually might feel the cold water, and his heartbeat actually might increase.

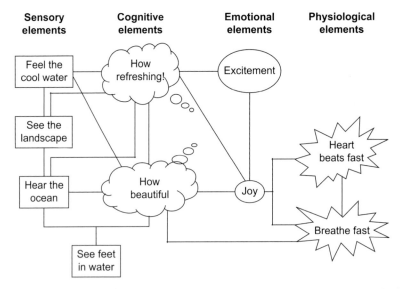

Fig. 1. Schematic presentation of a hypothetical sensory-perceptual representation including sensory, cognitive, emotional, and physiologic elements. The network represents a child's memory of a day on a beach during a holiday.

Like autobiographic representations, the sensory-perceptual representations of past events probably are not stored in a single brain structure. Neuroimaging studies suggest the complex involvement of the areas considered responsible for visuospatial processing and emotion (the limbic structures, especially the posterior cingulated, including the surrounding cortex and the occipital and parietal cortex) and for preparation for action (motor cortex) in the storage of sensory-perceptual representations [42].

There is good evidence that the amygdala plays a key role in the encoding and retrieval of highly arousing events, whether positive (exciting) or negative (frightening) [43,44]. Research on "flashbulb memories" [45] contributed to the knowledge about sensory-perceptual memory representations. Flashbulb memories are vivid and long-lasting memories of photographic quality about the environmental conditions of a person learning of a significant public event such as the terrorist attacks of September 11, 2001. The elevated arousal in this situation seems to support the encoding of a lasting sensory-perceptual representation of the situation. Recently it was shown that the amygdala is a key structure for the recall of flashbulb memories related to the September 11, 2001 terrorist attacks, at least for the persons who had been close to the event itself [46]. These findings fit well with animal research on fear conditioning, showing that the amygdala is the key structure for the learning associations between sensory stimuli and fear responses [47,48]. The effects of fear conditioning may be based on sensory-perceptual representations of the learning situation. Because the sensory and cognitive outputs of these memories cannot be studied with animal research, researchers have concentrated on the physiologic and behavioral responses to conditioned fear cues.

The effects of trauma on memory

Traumatic events are characterized by a massive threat to the victim requiring the immediate activation of the body in the form of an alarm response. Within seconds, the brain triggers the secretion of stress hormones, including the catecholamines norepinephrine and epinephrine. In combination with other immediate effects of sympathetic nervous activation, this response prepares the body system for a rapid fight-or-flight response. More slowly, peaking around 20 minutes after this rapid reaction, the hormonal messenger corticotropin, secreted by the pituitary gland, has traveled to the adrenal cortex, which releases the stress hormone cortisol that modulates a series of additional functions, including an increase in blood sugar level. The stress hormones travel back to the brain where they dock on receptors that are particularly dense in the hippocampus and dramatically modulate memory formation and consolidation [49]. In general, exposure to glucocorticoids (the stress hormone in rodents corresponding to human cortisol) increases the activity of the hippocampus, but the activity declines dramatically as soon as a certain threshold is exceeded. Under very high levels of stress and under chronic stress, the functioning of the hippocampus is impaired severely. At least in rodents [50,51], but probably also in primates [52], very high doses of adrenal steroids can cause permanent atrophy of the hippocampus.

Unlike the hippocampus, which shows decreased functioning under high levels of stress, the activity of the amygdala is enhanced as stress increases [53]. This enhanced activity also is caused by stress hormones [54,55]. A recent study with rats showed that whereas chronic stress induced dendritic atrophy in the hippocampus, the dendritic arborization of neurons in the amygdala was enhanced in the same condition [56]. The dissociation of amygdala and hippocampal functions during high levels of stress could be confirmed in humans. Using functional MRI and simultaneous skin conductance response measures, Williams and colleagues [57] demonstrated that amygdala networks were active only during the elaboration of arousing stimuli, whereas hippocampus activity occurred only in the absence of arousing stimuli.

The stress effects on amygdala and hippocampus affect the memory representations of the traumatic events. On one hand, the increased amygdala activity leads to an excessive sensory-perceptual representation of the event that has also been called "fear structure" [58]. As a result of the excessive amygdala activity during extreme stress, a fear structure differs from representations of normal events in several ways. First, the fear structures encoded during a traumatic event are unusually large and cover a wide variety of single items. As a consequence, they can be activated easily, because many environmental cues resemble the items in the fear structure. Second, interconnections between the single elements are unusually strong. Fig. 2 shows an example of a fear structure of a Sri Lankan child who has experienced both war and tsunami. As shown in the figure, multiple traumatic events can become part of a single fear structure because they share common elements like fear and physiologic arousal.

Because of the strong interconnection of items, the activation of only a few elements is sufficient to activate the whole structure, and this activation is difficult to control. The activation of the fear structure is experienced as an intrusive sensory, emotional, and physiologic re-experiencing of the traumatic event, the key symptom of PTSD. As a consequence, traumatized persons learn to prevent the activation of the structure by avoiding cues that remind them of the traumatic event. They must avoid both internal and external cues, so they try not to think about the even, try not to talk about it, and try to keep away from persons and places that remind them of the event. Eventually, the person acquires a pattern of avoidance behavior, another characteristic of PTSD.

Whereas extreme stress causes an excessive sensory-perceptual representation of the traumatic event, stress impairs the functioning of the hippocampus and the elaboration of an autobiographical representation. As a result, the traumatic event does not seem to be clearly represented as

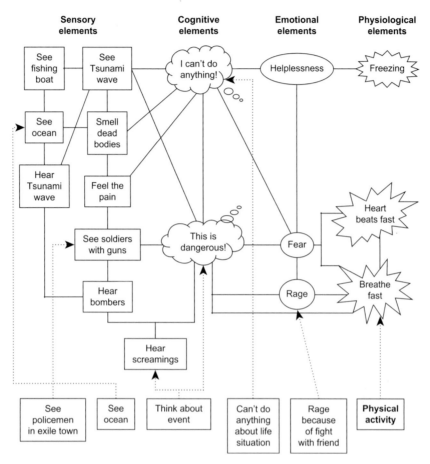

Fig. 2. Schematic presentation of a hypothetical sensory-perceptual representation of a traumatic event (fear structure) of a girl from Northern Sri Lanka. The network represents the memory of the Tsunami disaster mixed with war memories. The boxes below indicate environmental stimuli with the potential to activate the representation.

a specific event, and it does not seem to be clearly positioned in a lifetime period. Because a good autobiographical organization is necessary to narrate an event, the distortion in autobiographical memory leads to the failure of patients to talk about their traumatic experiences. In addition, the antagonism of the declarative and nondeclarative memory representations causes a distorted quality of retrieval of traumatic memory. The recollection of normal events usually is accompanied by the perception of subjective time, which means that even during the in-depth mental imagery of a past event a person always feels that this event took place at a different time and place. In contrast, the mostly intrusive recollection of traumatic memory is ungrounded by the narrative and spatiotemporal contextual anchors that tie ordinary experience to reality. Traumatic memories are disturbing, because of the direct fear they evoke and also because of their strangeness [36]. Lacking the autobiographical context, the intrusive memories are accompanied by the sensation of current threat, even though the event might have happened several years ago at a place very far away [30].

Taken together, the characteristic of traumatic memory is twofold. On the one hand, a person has very vivid recollections, including many sensory details. Despite the detailed representation of the memory, however, it is very difficult for the victim to narrate the event. Consistent with this assumption, several studies have shown that traumatic memory is qualitatively different from everyday memory [59]. Traumatic memory is more dominated by sensory elements and is highly distressing and repetitive, whereas the narrations are more fragmented [60]. In addition, Jones and co-workers [61] showed that disorganization of the narration and a dominance of sensory elements in the trauma memory immediately after the event predict the development of chronic PTSD.

Recovery from trauma: role of the supervising structure

Although most people react with an intensive emotional upheaval, including intrusive symptoms, immediately after a traumatic event, only a minority develops chronic PTSD. The recovery from acute stress symptoms is a normal process. In an influential account of emotional processing, Foa and Kozak [58] suggested that emotional processing involves the modification of the original fear structure. Research into fear conditioning has challenged this view. Several investigators have shown that extinction of fear responses usually does not change the original stimulus-fear associations, because the original fear response can be reinstated easily in a context different from the context of extinction learning. Instead, extinction probably occurs through the inhibition of the fear response by cortical areas, especially the medial prefrontal cortex [48]. Pathways from the prefrontal cortex to the amygdala allow the modification of a fear response, depending on the evaluation of the stimulus in the current environmental context. Recently, Shin and colleagues [62,63] showed that during symptom provocation (script-driven imagery), as well as during unspecific emotional stimulation, patients who had PTSD showed decreased activity in the medial prefrontal region but increased amygdala activity. In addition, amygdala activity correlated negatively with medial prefrontal activity and correlated positively with symptom severity. These findings indicate that persons who recovered from trauma symptoms can rely on an effective prefrontal mechanism to inhibit the activity of the amygdala-related fear structure. Animal research supports this view, because fear extinction depends on the activity of medial prefrontal areas rather than on changing amygdala-dependent associations [64–66], and sustained fear extinction requires memory consolidation in prefrontal areas involving protein synthesis [67].

Brewin [27] suggested that recovery from trauma symptoms depends on the availability of declarative autobiographical memory of the stimulus. This contextual knowledge is necessary to identify the intrusive flash of a fear structure after a trauma reminder as a memory process relating to past event rather than an indication of current threat. After a traumatic event, however, declarative knowledge, especially autobiographical knowledge that could offer information about the context of the feared stimulus, is fragmented or even absent. In this conceptualization, recovery from initial intrusive symptoms after a stressful event is the result of active emotional regulation rather than automatic extinction of fear responses. Recent imaging studies have shown that activity of the prefrontal brain structures correlate with active emotion regulation (eg, cognitive re-evaluation) [68–70] and with the inhibition of amygdala activity [69]. Furthermore, these structures overlap with areas responsible for extinction of conditioned responses [71]. These structures are key candidates for a supervisory structure that can control the activity of a fear structure, depending on the evaluation of the current situation and the memory content.

Traumatic memory in children

Episodic memory begins at the age of about 2 years, as soon as the children acquire a cognitive sense of self [72]. Theories of cognitive development suggest that early episodic memory is dominated by nondeclarative knowledge and contains little elaborate information about context and meaning [73]. Whereas sensory-perceptual representation can be established very early in life, fully functioning autobiographic memory depends on the development of a variety of cognitive functions, including mental concepts, temporal concepts, self-representations, language representations, and narrative structure [74]. In healthy children most of these structures have evolved sufficiently at the age of 5 years [32,74]. Because traumatic stress can affect a variety of brain structures during development [75], it is reasonable to assume that development of episodic memory may be delayed in children who grow up in stressful conditions. As a consequence, the memory theory outlined previously cannot be adapted unconditionally to children below the age of 5 years. In addition, the phenomenology of symptoms in traumatized preschool children differs to some extent from that in older children [76], and approaches to treatment must be adapted for these children [77].

Because of ethical concerns, there is a lack of research on the neurophysiology of trauma in children. In particular, there is no symptom-provocation study involving children. Some findings on traumatic memories do correspond with the neurocognitive theory, however. Recently, Kenardy and co-workers [78] examined children's trauma narratives in the aftermath of a traumatic event (4–7 weeks) and the presence of PTSD symptoms 6 months later. The authors found that temporal disorganization, but not absence of emotion, was associated with the presence of PTSD symptoms at a later stage. On the other hand, dissociative themes in the trauma narratives showed a weak link with the development of subsequent PTSD. These outcomes support the notion that in children, as well as in adults, traumatic memories might be characterized by a lack of coherent autobiographic information and, at the same time, by a dominant network of sensory and emotional elements.

In a recent longitudinal study [79], children who had a history of maltreatment underwent a variety of clinical evaluations at different time points over a period of 12 to 18 months. The study showed that the severity of PTSD symptoms as well as cortisol levels at baseline predicted hippocampal reduction. Even though additional studies are warranted to confirm these pilot data, the results of this study suggest an association among hippocampal changes, PTSD symptoms, and cortisol levels in traumatized children.

Consequences for treatment

In accordance with the neurocognitive theory of PTSD, the main goal of therapy could be the construction of a consistent declarative (autobiographic) representation of the traumatic event. Immediately after the fear structure has been activated by a reminder of a traumatic event, this declarative representation can provide the supervisory structure with the information that the activity of the fear structure is only a memory recollection and does not indicate a current threat. In turn, the supervisory structure can inhibit the activity of the fear structure. Consistent with this assumption, research on trauma treatment indicates that the construction of declarative trauma memory seems to be important for successful treatment. The exposure therapy developed by Foa and colleagues [25] has proven to be one of the most successful treatment approaches for PTSD. In exposure therapy for PTSD, the patient is instructed to talk about the traumatic experience repeatedly. Initial formulations of the theory of exposure therapy were based on fear extinction, but recent analyses of the treatment process support the importance of constructing autobiographic knowledge. In particular, it has been demonstrated that patients who manage to construct a coherent narration of the event during exposure therapy profit most from treatment [80].

The main focus of therapy should be on the part of the memory that is most fragmented in autobiography and is represented most intensively within the sensory-perceptual representations. To form a consistent autobiographic narration of this moment, the sensory-perceptual representation inevitably is activated, because it provides detailed knowledge about the event that is not yet available in declarative structures. The autobiographic representation should cover the most salient stimuli of the sensory-perceptual representation with the highest probability of eliciting intrusive symptoms. Because the activation of the sensory-perceptual representation always is accompanied by the emotional reactions coded in this structure, a high emotional involvement is necessary for therapy [81]. The task of a therapist is to encourage the activation of painful memories and to prevent the use of the patient's habitual strategies to avoid or terminate the activation. At the same time, the therapist should support the patient in organizing the declarative memory related to the traumatic event by assisting the narration of the event within the patient's biography. Although the activation of the sensory-perceptual representation leads to a high emotional response, the increasing formation of autobiographical knowledge should lead to an increasing capability by the supervisory structure to inhibit the fear reactions. This effect can be observed as habituation of the emotional response. This principle guides the procedure of NET.

The procedure of narrative exposure therapy

NET has been developed for application in crisis and postconflict regions. This context poses several challenges for a treatment approach. Because in these countries relatively few professionals are available for a high number of affected people, the treatment must be short and pragmatic. It should be easy to learn and be effective even when provided by trained laypersons or paraprofessionals with no or minimal medical or psychologic backgrounds. It should be applicable across cultures and fit into the social and political background of the setting.

Most researchers who are working with refugees or under field conditions in disaster and war regions are aware that any psychologic intervention needs a firm context. Although PTSD may be the most prevailing mental health disorder in most populations affected by war and disaster, a specific treatment module should be integrated into a sustainable and comprehensive psychosocial or mental health program that includes a variety of interventions and a referral structure for medical conditions. NET can be a key treatment program within such a structure; however, the therapist should be prepared to encounter common conditions, such as ongoing child abuse, substance dependence, grief, and depression. In addition to trauma therapy, therapists should have learned to identify and understand these problems so as to provide assistance or referral to other sources of help.

For the treatment of PTSD, the authors have developed NET, which is based on principles of the theory outlined in the previous sections [9,26,82]. For NET, the classical form of trauma exposure therapy was adapted to meet the needs of clinically traumatized survivors of war and torture. The different variants of exposure therapy for PTSD usually target the worst traumatic event, assuming that this approach will lead to the best treatment outcome. Most victims of organized violence, war, and torture have experienced several traumatic events, however, and often it is impossible to identify the worst event before treatment. In addition, the fear networks of different traumatic events overlap, and it can be difficult to sort out the origin of different network items. To overcome this challenge, NET uses the chronicity of testimony therapy. Instead of defining a single event as a target for therapy, the patient constructs a narrative of his or her whole life, from birth to the present, while focusing on the detailed report of the traumatic experiences. NET has been adapted for the use with traumatized children and adolescents in a version called "KidNET" [83].

KidNET should not be applied without a formal assessment of the child or adolescent. The typical inclusion criterion for therapy is a diagnosis of PTSD. KidNET has not been studied sufficiently in patients who have current substance addiction and psychosis, so at present these patients should be excluded. KidNET is a short-term treatment approach that usually takes between 4 and 10 sessions of 90 to 120 minutes. Box 1 presents the key

---

Box 1. Interventions of KidNET in an eight-session format

Prerequisite
Structured psychologic assessment including diagnosis of PTSD, comprehensive list of traumatic events, context condition (family background, current threats and violence), and exclusion criteria (substance addiction, psychosis)

First session
Psychoeducation with child and caretaker
Informed consent by caretaker and child
Lifeline

Second session
Revisit lifeline
Start narration at birth

Third through seventh sessions
Revisit lifeline
Reread and correct the narration of the previous session
Continue narration with focus on traumatic events

Eighth session
Revisit lifeline and add symbols for hopes in the future
Reread whole narration and include hopes for the future
Sign and hand over the narration

After treatment
Follow-up examination about 3 months after treatment

interventions in KidNET as applied in an eight-session treatment. The procedure for KidNET is described in the NET manual [26].

First session: psychoeducation and lifeline

Any trauma-focused treatment including an exposure element requires high motivation in the child and a good and trustful relationship between the child and the therapist. Consequently, treatment never should be started without detailed psychoeducation of the child. Parental consent should be obtained, if possible, and parents should be included in the psychoeducational part of treatment. The education includes information about trauma symptoms, a simplified model of the memory theory, the implications for treatment, and a detailed explanation of the treatment procedure. The child and the caretaker should be prepared for the activation of memories from the past that might be painful and that they might want to avoid; they should know that the therapist will counteract this tendency. Depending on the child's age, different metaphors can be used to explain the memory theory. (One example is the metaphor of a cabinet that is so full and messy that items fall out of it. Constantly holding the doors and occasionally putting the items back might be one solution, but it would be better to open doors once and to sort the items systematically.) In KidNET, parents or caretakers are present only during the psychoeducational part of treatment. The rest of the treatment is conducted with the child alone (or with an interpreter if necessary), to allow the child to make his or her own report free of the influences of the parents or caretakers.

The next step in treatment is the lifeline procedure. The therapist presents a rope and explains to the child that it symbolizes his or her life, with the beginning of the rope marking the birth. The child is asked to lay the rope out on the floor, leaving a part of the rope unfolded to represent the future. The therapist then presents flowers and stones of different sizes and colors to the child and explains that the flowers represent happy moments in life, and the stones stand for bad experiences (eg, sad, fearful, or painful events). The therapist asks the child to place the flowers and stones along the lifeline to mark significant life events. The therapist assists the child in finding the right chronology of events. Because the aim of the procedure is to obtain a rough overview of the child's life rather than emotional disclosure, the child gives only a very short description—a headline—of each event. After all major events are represented on the lifeline, the child makes a drawing of this lifeline and writes the headline next to each symbol. Older children might prefer to take a photograph of the lifeline instead of drawing. The picture of the lifeline serves as an important tool for knowing where the key moments in the child's life are located. During treatment, more events (more stones and flowers) might be revealed, and the picture can be corrected accordingly.

The second session

At the start of each session, the child revisits the picture of the lifeline. Then the child starts to narrate his or her life. The therapist takes care of the chronology of events and starts the procedure with direct questions like "Where were you born?" and "Who are your parents?" The narration should focus both on factual background information and on vividly recorded emotional events. In fortunate cases, the first emotional event can be a positive event that should be explored in much detail, using the same techniques used for traumatic events to teach the child the procedure of chronologic and emotional narration. The therapist writes down the narration as a first-person account in the past tense. The start of a narration of a 12-year-old Sudanese boy could look like this:

> I grew up in Yei. We were a large family. My father had four wives by then. And he had 11 children, four girls and seven boys. My father was a rich man. He had goats and cattle. So there was a competition among the children. My father preferred the children of another wife. Me, my brother Nicolas, and my sister Sylvia were among the neglected ones. But I remember well, when we were children, we enjoyed playing in the field while the parents were uprooting cassava.

The following sessions

At the start of the following sessions the therapist takes some time to explore how the child has been faring between the sessions. This understanding is particularly important, because some children have more intrusive symptoms and nightmares following the initial NET sessions. The therapist explains to the child that this phenomenon is an indication of emotional processing and that the child should not be afraid of this occurrence. After the therapist and the child have indicated the current state of therapy at the lifeline, the therapist asks the child whether he or she wants to modify the lifeline: perhaps the child has remembered additional major events. The therapist then rereads the narration that was written down in the previous session. The therapist instructs the child to be very attentive, to imagine the events again, and to correct the story. Usually, the child adds some information or even new events. The therapist is aware of uncertainties in chronology and resolves these issues with the child. The narration then continues until the current situation.

The last session

In the last treatment session, the child is asked to lay down his or her lifeline again. This time, the lifeline is extended with flowers to represent the hopes and wishes for the future. The therapist reads the narration to the child one last time and adds the hopes and wishes for the future. At the end, all persons who were involved in the treatment (ie, the child, the therapist, and the interpreter) sign the final document. The therapist discusses with the child the further use of the testimony and hands one copy to the child, who is free to do with it whatever he or she wants. The therapist, however, explains the potential dangers involved in politically sensitive cases.

Narrating traumatic events

The most important and most sensitive element of KidNET is the narration of the traumatic events. Within KidNET, a traumatic event should be narrated only using a very directive approach that requires some skills and a clear understanding of the neurocognitive theory outlined earlier.

Even though most traumatic events should be predictable in the narration, because they are represented as stones on the lifeline, the therapist should be aware of events that turn out to be very dramatic during the narration or events that have been left out on the lifeline. Several indicators show that the child might be approaching a traumatic event in his or her story. The child might show some observable activation of the fear structure (ie, become nervous, tense, and fearful). At the same time, the child might want to avoid the narration by getting impatient and rushing through a period of life or by presenting an urgent need for a break. At this moment the therapist must make a clear decision whether to go explore the event in detail or to postpone the continuation to the next session, because the narration of a traumatic event usually requires about 1 hour and must not be interrupted. As soon as the therapist decides to explore the event, he or she must be very directive in the exploration to keep a clear chronology. Usually, the story is fragmented and dominated by single perceptions of the worst moment of the event. The therapist directs the child to start the event at the beginning, including background information about the temporal and spatial context of the event. The event is then explored in slow motion, in much detail, always keeping the chronology of the event clear. By asking the child direct questions ("What did you see?") and making probing observations ("I can see that you are trembling now. Did you feel like trembling then?"), the therapist makes sure that all aspects of the memory—including "cold" facts as well as "hot" elements from the fear structure—are present at each step of the story. In this way, elements from the fear structure (sensory perceptions, cognitions, emotions, and physiologic responses) are anchored in the framework of a chronologic life event that is based in autobiographic memory. As a consequence, a habituation of emotional responses can be observed during the narration. The child will notice a decrease in fear and perhaps even some feelings of relief. The therapist always should be aware of the increasing and decreasing states of arousal and fear in the child and never should end a session while the child is still highly aroused and occupied by memories of the traumatic event. After the narration of a traumatic event, the child might want to discuss some aspects of the meaning of this event. The therapist can use methods from cognitive therapy to modify maladaptive assumptions and conclusions, especially when the child feels high levels of shame and guilt.

The use of illustrative media

The main tool of narrative exposure is language. Even though autobiographical memory processes, including narrative language, are reasonably well established at the age of 5 years [74], children need more assistance than adults in creating their autobiographic memory, especially for memories that happened before the age of 5 years. Although the child's level of language development at the time of encoding influences the extent to which events can be reported verbally, children at the age of 5 years can provide a brief verbal report of a stressful experience that happened already at the age of 3 years [84]. However, Children, including very young ones, can provide additional information to their verbal report if they are given the opportunity to illustrate their memories [85].

In addition to language development, the child's emotional and cognitive capabilities must be taken into account in trauma treatment [86]. Unlike other treatment approaches for traumatized children, KidNET does not contain a module of training in emotion regulation or affective coping. Nevertheless, the therapist must be aware of the individual child's state of emotional and cognitive development. Most school-aged children can understand at least the basic emotions of fear, anger, sadness, and happiness and can infer the causes of the emotional states [87]. Children's narrations of emotional events usually contain few references to emotions, however [88]. The child–parent communication is the main medium of emotional development. Because child–parent interactions can be severely impaired in traumatized children, many of them present with a marked delay in emotional development.

Because of these developmental factors, the therapist must be aware of the emotional and cognitive capabilities of the individual child. Often the therapist must assist directly in creating an understandable narration. For example, the therapist must be aware of a child's difficulties in classifying and verbalizing emotions and teach the child about basic emotions. Many children have difficulties judging the event that have happened to them, especially in cases of taboo and shameful events such as sexual victimization. A lack of knowledge about children's rights and the context of violence can leave them with a lack of understanding of their own biography. The therapist can educate the child directly about the context of the particular form of violence and can acknowledge the injustice that has happened to him or her.

The use of creative media can compensate for children's difficulties with memory and reporting by providing a chain of retrieval cues, a structure for the child's narrative [89], and assistance in understanding and verbalizing emotions [90]. Therapists, however, must be be very cautious not to be suggestive when using illustrative material to avoid the installation of false memories [91].

KidNET involves the use of specific creative media that aid in retrieval of memory and help the narration of a past event. Such tools are the lifeline, drawing, and re-enactment using body positioning or playing out (eg, using little figures or toys) of key moments of the traumatic event. The use of illustrative material always is accompanied by verbal narration. While drawing or playing, the child is encouraged to explain his or her drawing or activity, and the therapist verbalizes along empathically. The dialogue is guided by the rationale of NET treatment: cognitions, emotions, and physiologic and sensory memory within the flow of chronology. For example, the drawing of a scene might be accompanied like this: "I can see a little boy with a red T-shirt by the side of the road here. Is this you? Ah sure, I can recognize your dark hair. Do you remember what you were thinking in that moment as you stood there? How do you feel now you are drawing this?" Body positioning is a different technique that requires the child to assume the position he or she had during the traumatic event. Because the kinesthetic perception is part of the sensory-perceptual representation of the event, this technique might help trigger other hot memories of the event. Because this method can be very powerful in triggering emotions, the therapist should be careful to stay in close contact with the child and to keep assisting in narrating the event.

Basic rules

The treatment of traumatized children requires several ground rules for the basic behavior and attitude of the therapist. The ground rules (security, control, predictability, physical integrity, acceptance, empathy, congruence, and confidentiality) are explained in more detail in the manual [26]. The main challenge for the therapist is to overcome his or her own avoidance of strong emotions. As a consequence, especially in conflict regions, a processing of the practitioner's traumatic experiences is a key element of NET training.

Outcome of narrative exposure therapy in children

So far, one case report and two randomized, controlled trials using NET with adults have been published [9,82,92]. In general, these studies with Sudanese refugees in Uganda and with survivors of political violence in Romania showed a clinically significant reduction in PTSD symptoms and greater effectiveness than supportive counseling and psychoeducation only. Treatment effects have been maintained for up to 1 year, and the data show that within the first year after treatment the symptoms continue to decline in comparison with the post-test administered immediately after therapy. Three case reports and a small case series on KidNET used to treat war-traumatized children living in a Ugandan refugee camp have appeared in print [83,93]. In meantime, controlled studies have been completed. A randomized, controlled trial with traumatized refugee children in Germany showed that children who received KidNET had a large decrease in PTSD in comparison with children on the waiting list. A controlled study with children and adolescents orphaned in the Rwandan genocide demonstrated lasting and rather strong effects. Trials in Sri Lanka proved that KidNET can be disseminated effectively to teachers who then could treat war-traumatized children successfully. Thus there is increasing evidence that KidNET significantly reduces symptoms of PTSD even in severely war-traumatized children. KidNET also seems to have a significant effect on the symptoms of depression and on suicidal ideation. These findings show that KidNET is a feasible, pragmatic, and effective tool for the short-term treatment of child and adolescent victims of war and violence.

References

[1] Kaldor M. New and old wars: organized violence in a global era. London: Blackwell; 1999.
[2] International Federation of Red Cross and Red Crescent Societies. World disasters report 2004. Geneva: International Federation of Red Cross and Red Crescent Societies.
[3] Catani C, Jacob N, Schauer E, et al. When family violence adds to war and natural disaster: mental health of children living under extreme stress in Sri-Lanka BMC Psychiatry, in press.
[4] Ehntholt KA, Yule W. Practitioner review: assessment and treatment of refugee children and adolescents who have experienced war-related trauma. J Child Psychol Psychiatry 2006;47: 1197–210.
[5] Saigh PA. The development of posttraumatic stress disorder following four different types of traumatization. Behav Res Ther 1991;29:213–6.
[6] Schaal S, Elbert T. Ten years after the genocide: trauma confrontation and posttraumatic stress in Rwandan adolescents. J Trauma Stress 2006;19:95–105.
[7] Elbert T, Huschka B, Schauer E, et al. Trauma-related impairment in children—an epidemiological survey in Sri Lankan provinces affected by two decades of civil war and unrest. Child Abuse Negl, in press.
[8] Neuner F, Schauer E, Catani C, et al. Post tsunami stress: a study of posttraumatic stress disorder in children living in three severely affected regions in Sri Lanka. J Trauma Stress 2006;19:339–47
[9] Neuner F, Schauer M, Klaschik C, et al. A comparison of narrative exposure therapy, supportive counseling, and psychoeducation for treating posttraumatic stress disorder in an African refugee settlement. J Consult Clin Psychol 2004;72:579–87.
[10] Meiser-Stedman R, Yule W, Smith P, et al. Acute stress disorder and posttraumatic stress disorder in children and adolescents involved in assaults or motor vehicle accidents. Am J Psychiatry 2005;162:1381–3.
[11] Sack WH, Him C, Dickason D. Twelve-year follow-up study of Khmer youths who suffered massive war trauma as children. J Am Acad Child Adolesc Psychiatry 1999;38: 1173–9.
[12] Bolton P, Bass J, Betancourt T, et al. Interventions for depression symptoms among adolescent survivors of war and displacement in northern Uganda: a randomized controlled trial. JAMA 2007;298:519–27.

[13] Cohen JA, Deblinger E, Mannarino AP, et al. A multisite, randomized controlled trial for children with sexual abuse-related PTSD symptoms. J Am Acad Child Adolesc Psychiatry 2004;43:393–402.

[14] Stein BD, Jaycox LH, Kataoka SH, et al. A mental health intervention for schoolchildren exposed to violence: a randomized controlled trial. JAMA 2003;290:603–11.

[15] Stallard P. Psychological interventions for post-traumatic reactions in children and young people: a review of randomised controlled trials. Clin Psychol Rev 2006;26: 895–911.

[16] Deblinger E, Steer RA, Lippmann J. Two-year follow-up study of cognitive behavioral therapy for sexually abused children suffering post-traumatic stress symptoms. Child Abuse Negl 1999;23:1371–8.

[17] Smith P, Dyregrov A, Yule W, et al. Children and war: teaching recovery techniques. Bergen, Norway: Children and War Foundation; 2000.

[18] Saltzman WR, Layne CM, Steinberg AM, et al. Developing a culturally and ecologically sound intervention program for youth exposed to war and terrorism. Child Adolesc Psychiatr Clin N Am 2003;12:319–42, x.

[19] Giannopoulou I, Dikaiakou A, Yule W. Cognitive-behavioural group intervention for PTSD symptoms in children following the Athens 1999 earthquake: a pilot study. Clin Child Psychol Psychiatry 2006;11:543–53.

[20] Goenjian AK, Karayan I, Pynoos RS, et al. Outcome of psychotherapy among early adolescents after trauma. Am J Psychiatry 1997;154:536–42.

[21] Chemtob CM, Nakashima JP, Hamada RS. Psychosocial intervention for postdisaster trauma symptoms in elementary school children: a controlled community field study. Arch Pediatr Adolesc Med 2002;156:211–6.

[22] Ehntholt KA, Smith P, Yule W. School-based cognitive-behavioural therapy group intervention for refugee children who have experienced war-related trauma. Clin Child Psychol Psychiatry 2005;10:235–50.

[23] Thabet AA, Vostanis P, Karim K. Group crisis intervention for children during ongoing war conflict. Eur Child Adolesc Psychiatry 2005;14:262–9.

[24] Cienfuegos J, Monelli C. The testimony of political repression as a therapeutic instrument. Am J Orthopsychiatry 1983;53:43–51.

[25] Foa EB, Rothbaum BO. Treating the trauma of rape: cognitive-behavioral therapy for PTSD. Treatment manuals for practitioners. New York; Guilford Press: 1998.

[26] Schauer M, Neuner F, Elbert T. Narrative exposure therapy—a short term intervention for traumatic stress disorders after war, terror or torture. Seattle; Hogrefe: 2005.

[27] Brewin CR. A cognitive neuroscience account of posttraumatic stress disorder and its treatment. Behav Res Ther 2001;39:373–93.

[28] Brewin CR, Holmes EA. Psychological theories of posttraumatic stress disorder. Clin Psychol Rev 2003;23:339–76.

[29] Dalgleish T. Cognitive approaches to posttraumatic stress disorder: the evolution of multirepresentational theorizing. Psychol Bull 2004;130:228–60.

[30] Ehlers A, Clark DM. A cognitive model of posttraumatic stress disorder. Behav Res Ther 2000;38:319–45.

[31] Tulving E. Episodic memory and common sense: how far apart? Philos Trans R Soc Lond B Biol Sci 2001;356:1505–15.

[32] Howe ML, Toth S, Cicchetti D. Memory and developmental psychopathology. In: Cicchetti D, Cohen D, editors. Developmental psychopathology. Developmental neuroscience, vol. 2. 2nd edition. New York: Wiley; 2006. p. 106–25.

[33] Squire LR. Declarative and nondeclarative memory: multiple brain systems supporting learning and memory. In: Schacter DL, Tulving E, editors. Memory systems 1994. Cambridge (MA): MIT Press; 1994. p. 207–28.

[34] Conway MA, Pleydell-Pearce CW. The construction of autobiographical memories in the self-memory system. Psychol Rev 2000;107:261–88.

[35] Brewin CR, Dalgleish T, Joseph S. A dual representation theory of posttraumatic stress disorder. Psychol Rev 1996;103:670–86.

[36] Metcalve J, Jacobs W. A "hot-system/cool-system" view of memory under stress. PTSD Research Quarterly 1996;7:1–3.

[37] Dudai Y. The neurobiology of consolidations, or, how stable is the engram? Annu Rev Psychol 2004;55:51–86.

[38] Shastri L. Episodic memory and cortico-hippocampal interactions. Trends Cogn Sci 2002;6: 162–8.

[39] McClelland JL, McNaughton BL, O'Reilly RC. Why there are complementary learning systems in the hippocampus and neocortex: insights from the successes and failures of connectionist models of learning and memory. Psychol Rev 1995;102:419–57.

[40] Conway MA. Sensory-perceptual episodic memory and its context: autobiographical memory. Philos Trans R Soc Lond B Biol Sci 2001;356:1375–84.

[41] Lang P. A bio-informational theory of emotional imagery. Psychophysiology 1979;16: 495–512.

[42] Bremner JD. Neuroimaging studies in post-traumatic stress disorder. Curr Psychiatry Rep 2002;4:254–63.

[43] Kensinger EA. Remembering emotional experiences: the contribution of valence and arousal. Rev Neurosci 2004;15:241–51.

[44] Canli T, Zhao Z, Brewer J, et al. Event-related activation in the human amygdala associates with later memory for individual emotional experience. J Neurosci 2000;20:RC99.

[45] Brown R, Kulik J. Flashbulb memories. Cognition 1977;5:73–99.

[46] Sharot T, Martorella EA, Delgado MR, et al. How personal experience modulates the neural circuitry of memories of September 11. Proc Natl Acad Sci U S A 2007;104:389–94.

[47] LeDoux JE. Emotion: clues from the brain. Annu Rev Psychol 1995;46:209–35.

[48] LeDoux JE. Emotion circuits in the brain. Annu Rev Neurosci 2000;23:155–84.

[49] Miller MM, McEwen BS. Establishing an agenda for translational research on PTSD. Ann N Y Acad Sci 2006;1071:294–312.

[50] Kim JJ, Yoon KS. Stress: metaplastic effects in the hippocampus. Trends Neurosci 1998;21: 505–9.

[51] McEwen BS. Stress and hippocampal plasticity. Annu Rev Neurosci 1999;22:105–22.

[52] Sapolsky RM, Uno H, Rebert CS, et al. Hippocampal damage associated with prolonged glucocorticoid exposure in primates. J Neurosci 1990;10:2897–902.

[53] Pitman RK, Shalev AY, Orr SP. Posttraumatic stress disorder: emotion, conditioning and memory. In: Gazzaniga MS, editor. The new cognitive neurosciences. Cambridge (MA): MIT Press; 2000. p. 72–96.

[54] Duvarci S, Pare D. Glucocorticoids enhance the excitability of principal basolateral amygdala neurons. J Neurosci 2007;27:4482–91.

[55] Debiec J, LeDoux JE. Noradrenergic signaling in the amygdala contributes to the reconsolidation of fear memory: treatment implications for PTSD. Ann N Y Acad Sci 2006;1071: 521–4.

[56] Vyas A, Mitra R, Shankaranarayana Rao BS, et al. Chronic stress induces contrasting patterns of dendritic remodeling in hippocampal and amygdaloid neurons. J Neurosci 2002;22:6810–8.

[57] Williams LM, Phillips ML, Brammer MJ, et al. Arousal dissociates amygdala and hippocampal fear responses: evidence from simultaneous fMRI and skin conductance recording. Neuroimage 2001;14:1070–9.

[58] Foa EB, Kozak MJ. Emotional processing of fear: exposure to corrective information. Psychol Bull 1986;99:20–35.

[59] Brewin CR. Autobiographical memory for trauma: update on four controversies. Memory 2007;15:227–48.

[60] Harvey AG, Bryant RA. A qualitative investigation of the organization of traumatic memories. Br J Clin Psychol 1999;38:401–5.

[61] Jones C, Harvey AG, Brewin CR. The organisation and content of trauma memories in survivors of road traffic accidents. Behav Res Ther 2007;45:151–62.

[62] Shin LM, Orr SP, Carson MA, et al. Regional cerebral blood flow in the amygdala and medial prefrontal cortex during traumatic imagery in male and female Vietnam veterans with PTSD. Arch Gen Psychiatry 2004;61:168–76.

[63] Shin LM, Wright CI, Cannistraro PA, et al. A functional magnetic resonance imaging study of amygdala and medial prefrontal cortex responses to overtly presented fearful faces in post-traumatic stress disorder. Arch Gen Psychiatry 2005;62:273–81.

[64] Milad MR, Quirk GJ. Neurons in medial prefrontal cortex signal memory for fear extinction. Nature 2002;420:70–4.

[65] Quirk GJ, Gehlert DR. Inhibition of the amygdala: key to pathological states? Ann N Y Acad Sci 2003;985:263–72.

[66] Quirk GJ, Likhtik E, Pelletier JG, et al. Stimulation of medial prefrontal cortex decreases the responsiveness of central amygdala output neurons. J Neurosci 2003;23:8800–7.

[67] Santini E, Ge H, Ren K, et al. Consolidation of fear extinction requires protein synthesis in the medial prefrontal cortex. J Neurosci 2004;24:5704–10.

[68] Hariri AR, Mattay VS, Tessitore A, et al. Neocortical modulation of the amygdala response to fearful stimuli. Biol Psychiatry 2003;53:494–501.

[69] Ochsner KN, Bunge SA, Gross JJ, et al. Rethinking feelings: an FMRI study of the cognitive regulation of emotion. J Cogn Neurosci 2002;14:1215–29.

[70] Phan KL, Fitzgerald DA, Nathan PJ, et al. Neural substrates for voluntary suppression of negative affect: a functional magnetic resonance imaging study. Biol Psychiatry 2005;57:210–9.

[71] Phelps EA. Emotion and cognition: insights from studies of the human amygdala. Annu Rev Psychol 2006;57:27–53.

[72] Howe ML. The fate of early memories: developmental science and the retention of childhood experiences. Washington; American Psychological Association.

[73] Brainerd CJ, Reyna VF. Fuzzy-trace theory: dual processes in memory, reasoning, and cognitive neuroscience. Adv Child Dev Behav 2001;28:41–100.

[74] Nelson K, Fivush R. The emergence of autobiographical memory: a social cultural developmental theory. Psychol Rev 2004;111:486–511.

[75] Teicher MH, Andersen SL, Polcari A, et al. Developmental neurobiology of childhood stress and trauma. Psychiatr Clin North Am 2002;25:397–426, vii–viii.

[76] Scheeringa MS, Zeanah CH, Myers L, et al. New findings on alternative criteria for PTSD in preschool children. J Am Acad Child Adolesc Psychiatry 2003;42:561–70.

[77] Scheeringa MS, Salloum A, Arnberger RA, et al. Feasibility and effectiveness of cognitive-behavioral therapy for posttraumatic stress disorder in preschool children: two case reports. J Trauma Stress 2007;20:631–6.

[78] Kenardy J, Smith A, Spence SH, et al. Dissociation in children's trauma narratives: an exploratory investigation. J Anxiety Disord 2007;21:456–66.

[79] Carrion VG, Weems CF, Reiss AL. Stress predicts brain changes in children: a pilot longitudinal study on youth stress, posttraumatic stress disorder, and the hippocampus. Pediatrics 2007;119:509–16.

[80] Foa EB, Molnar C, Cashman L. Change in rape narratives during exposure therapy for posttraumatic stress disorder. J Trauma Stress 1995;4:675–90.

[81] Jaycox LH, Foa EB, Morral AR. Influence of emotional engagement and habituation on exposure therapy for PTSD. J Consult Clin Psychol 1998;66:185–92.

[82] Neuner F, Schauer M, Elbert T, et al. A narrative exposure treatment as intervention in a Macedonia's refugee camp: a case report. J Behav Cogn Psychother 2002;30:205–9.

[83] Onyut LP, Neuner F, Schauer E, et al. Narrative exposure therapy as a treatment for child war survivors with posttraumatic stress disorder: two case reports and a pilot study in an African refugee settlement. BMC Psychiatry 2005;5.

[84] Peterson C, Rideout R. Memory for medical emergencies experienced by 1- and 2-year-olds. Dev Psychol 1998;34:1059–72.

[85] Driessnack M. Children's drawings as facilitators of communication: a meta-analysis. J Pediatr Nurs 2005;20:415–23.

[86] Salmon K, Bryant B. Posttraumatic stress disorder in children—the influence of developmental factors. Clin Psychol Rev 2002;22:163–88.

[87] Ashiabi GS. Promoting the emotional development of preschoolers. Early Child Educ J 2000;28:79–84.

[88] Fivush R. Children's memories of emotional events. In: Reisberg D, Hertel P, editors. Memory and emotion. Oxford (UK): Oxford University Press; 2003. p. 242–71.

[89] Gross J, Hayne H. Drawing facilitates children's verbal reports of emotionally laden events. J Exp Psychol Appl 1998;4:163–79.

[90] Wesson M, Salmon K. Drawin and showing: helping children to report emotionally laden events. Appl Cogn Psychol 2001;15:301–20.

[91] Brown DA, Pipe ME, Lewis C, et al. Supportive or suggestive: do human figure drawings help 5- to 7-year-old children to report touch? J Consult Clin Psychol 2007;75:33–42.

[92] Bichescu D, Neuner F, Schauer M, et al. Narrative exposure therapy for political imprisonment-related chronic posttraumatic stress disorder and depression. Behav Res Ther 2007;45: 2212–20.

[93] Schauer E, Neuner F, Elbert T, et al. Narrative exposure therapy in children: a case study. Intervention 2004;2:18–38.

ELSEVIER
SAUNDERS

Child Adolesc Psychiatric Clin N Am
17 (2008) 665–683

CHILD AND
ADOLESCENT
PSYCHIATRIC CLINICS
OF NORTH AMERICA

The Child Asylum Seeker: Psychological and Developmental Impact of Immigration Detention

Louise K. Newman, FRANZCP, PhD[a],*,
Zachary Steel, MPsychol(Clinical)[b]

[a]Perinatal and Infant Psychiatry, School of Medicine and Public Health Faculty of Health,
The University of Newcastle, Callaghan Campus, Locked Bag 1014, Wallsend,
New South Wales 2308, Australia
[b]Centre for Population Mental Health Research, Sydney South West Area Health Service and
Psychiatry Research and Teaching Unit School of Psychiatry, University of New South Wales,
Sydney, New South Wales, Australia

Child asylum seekers and policies of deterrence

The late twentieth century has witnessed an increase in the number of persons affected by war, persecution, and displacement. Significant numbers of adults and children have been exposed to trauma and violence during recent decades [1]. Children constitute a significant proportion of asylum-seeking and refugee populations worldwide and are particularly vulnerable to the effects of trauma, displacement, and loss.

At the end of 2005, of the 19 million persons of concern to the Office of the United Nations High Commissioner for Refugees (UNHCR), 12% were estimated to be less than 5 years of age, and 32% were children aged 6 to 17 years [2]. These figures represent a reduction from a peak of nearly 27 million persons in the mid 1990s [3]. The number of refugees in need of permanent resettlement far exceeds the number of places available from the 10 or so traditional countries that have formalized refugee resettlement programs [4]. Because most industrialized countries have no formal resettlement program, the main mechanism available to those seeking protection continues to be that of applying for political asylum. During the 10-year period from 1995 to 2004, 4.8 million asylum seekers sought protection directly

* Corresponding author.
E-mail address: louise.newman@newcastle.edu.au (L.K. Newman).

from industrialized countries, and 1.5 million were offered refugee or humanitarian protection.

The patterns of asylum seeking manifest over the previous 20 years have corresponded closely to global patterns of conflict and political unrest. Nevertheless, countries of the West have shown an increasing reluctance to provide protection to those seeking asylum, resorting instead to a range of measures of so-called "humane deterrence" [4,5]. By far the most effective of these strategies has been the increased focus on security (eg, national or regional border protection, the implementation of document and travel restrictions, and more recently interdiction at sea) to limit the flow of potential asylum seekers from conflict zones. Another important component of this policy has been the implementation of stringent administrative or judicial refugee assessment procedures with restricted access for appeal. Closely associated with this process has been the decision on the part of a number of countries not to hear refugee claims from individuals who have passed through countries where they might have been able to obtain effective protection. At a national level many countries have implemented various policies to limit or exclude asylum seekers from civil entitlements, such as health care, welfare, housing, and work rights. Public discourse regularly conflates issues of asylum and refugee protection with illegal migration, smuggling, and, more recently, terrorism [6,7]. Similarly, there has been little focus in public discourse on the high level of exposure to trauma (eg, organized violence, atrocities, sexual assault, and the death of immediate and extended family) experienced by asylum seekers, including entire families and children [4].

The increasingly harsh reception policies aimed at asylum seekers have a direct impact on children, because children, whether accompanied by parents or on their own, account for as many as half of all asylum seekers in the industrialized world [8]. Moreover, there has been a large rise in the number of unaccompanied and separated children applying for asylum in recent years. In 2003, for instance, 12,800 separated children applied for asylum in 28 industrialized countries [9].

The rights of child asylum seekers are protected by a range of international and regional conventions and declarations including the United Nations Convention on the Rights of the Child (UNCRC), the European Convention on Human Rights, the Geneva Convention, the International Covenant on Civil and Political Rights, and the International Covenant on Economic, Social and Cultural Rights. There can be little doubt that the range of restrictions being applied to asylum seekers is at odds with many of the protections enshrined in these conventions, including children's rights to protection, social participation, the living conditions necessary for the child's development, and the highest attainable standard of health. There seems, for instance, to be a clear association between the imposition of postmigration stressors and poor mental health outcomes [10–13].

Child asylum seekers have had a range of experiences that put them at high risk of psychological distress and the development of mental disorder. A 1996 study of refugee entrants in New South Wales, Australia, found that 25%, including children, had been subject to torture and trauma. Children had been the victims of persistent and long-term political repression with threats to themselves and their families. They had experienced loss of shelter and/or forced displacement from home. Some had witnessed murder and cruelty or had family members disappear. Children were particularly vulnerable in the face of separation from family and caregivers and were more likely to be abused and victimized in refugee camp situations. They suffered the effects of malnutrition, disease, and neglect [14]. Despite this evidence of risk, there are few specialist mental health and support services for asylum-seeking and refugee children, and the experience of immigration detention, applied to some groups of asylum seekers, is itself a risk factor for mental disorder [15].

Children and immigration detention: an international overview

Perhaps the most controversial policy in recent years has been the administrative application of immigration detention to certain categories of asylum seekers, including children, for all or part of the refugee determination process. The United States, the United Kingdom, Germany, Italy, and, until recently, Australia detain significant numbers of children for immigration-related matters [16,17]. The routine practice of detaining children, either alone or as part of a family group, seems to stand in conflict with the UNCRC, which stresses that detention of children should be used only as a measure of last resort and for the shortest appropriate period of time [18].

The treatment of child asylum seekers varies widely, and the use of immigration detention has been practiced in a manner that has been found to be arbitrary in several countries, raising issues of the status of human rights conventions and the capacity of states to override or ignore them. The British government, for instance, has formally entered a reservation to the UNCRC enabling children subject to immigration control to be excluded from human rights provisions. During 2006 it is estimated that some 1650 minors were subject to detention in the United Kingdom [19], a number slightly lower than in 2005, when 1850 children were held in United Kingdom immigration detention centers, 320 of whom were detained for more than 14 days [20]. Within the United States more than 5000 children are held in immigration detention on an annual basis [21], excluding the larger number of children that are intercepted and detained for short periods on the United States/Mexican border before repatriation [22]. In 2006 in Texas, the United States opened a 512-bed facility built especially for family detention [23], demonstrating an ongoing commitment to the detention of family groups in that country.

Australia emerges as a particularly important case example, with most information and research about the impact of immigration detention emerging from the experiences of children and families held for extended periods. In 1992, the Australian government instituted legislation mandating the detention of all undocumented noncitizens, including asylum seekers and their families. There was no mechanism for judicial review of detention, and no time limits were placed on the duration of detention. Despite recent policy changes and moves toward the community detention of children and families, mandatory detention of children remains enshrined in Australian law despite international conventions. The following section provides a detailed review of the Australian situation.

The Australian experience of mandatory detention

Australia was the first developed nation to introduce a policy of mandatory detention of all unauthorized arrivals coming by boat or without a valid entry visa. In 1994 an original 273-day time limit on detention was removed, allowing indefinite detention with no exemptions made for children or unaccompanied minors. The Australian High Court confirmed the power of the state to detain unlawful noncitizens indefinitely for the purposes of immigration control and ruled that immigration law took primacy over child welfare and protection legislation. The number of boat arrivals to Australian territories began to surge during 1999 as people-smuggling operations became established in Malaysia and Indonesia. A substantial proportion of arrivals included children: 2184 children arrived by boat during the 4-year period from July 1999 to June 2003. Pursuant to the policy of mandatory detention, all these children were placed in detention, for an average period of 9 months. The average length of detention later increased and reached 20 months by December 2003 [24].

Detention facilities were constructed in extremely remote desert regions of the country with minimal access to legal, health, and support services. Private contractors operated these facilities along the lines of penal institutions, with a focus on behavioral regulation and control. Minimal provisions were made to assess or address the health, mental health, or psychosocial needs of detainees despite evidence that many had experienced torture and trauma. The specific needs of children and adolescents were not considered; inadequate environments and limited play and educational opportunities were provided for young children [24]. The detention facilities have been the object of criticism in several Commissions of Inquiry that describe a culture of punishment, humiliating treatment of detainees, including children, and a failure to provide appropriate psychological support for high-risk populations. Children were noted to be particularly vulnerable, especially in the context of parental distress and depression, and to have been subject to maltreatment, such as being called by a number rather than by name. Children were exposed to repeated outbreaks of protest and a milieu that seemed to promote behaviors born of despair, such as self-harm and hunger strikes. The rate of completed suicides from 2001 to 2003 was comparable to that in other high-risk groups in detention, such as Australian indigenous peoples [25].

From the inception of the policy, mental health professionals raised clinical and ethical concerns regarding the impact of mandatory detention and particularly the impact of this policy on children [26,27]. Concerns were raised in the 1998 Australian Human Rights and Equal Opportunity Commission (HREOC) inquiry that prolonged detention resulted in depression and distress and was associated with suicidal behavior [28]. The 2004 HREOC inquiry heard evidence about the impact of prolonged detention on child development and mental health and determined that the detention of children was clearly detrimental to their mental health [24].

The negative outcome for children was seen as being related to the deprived conditions of the detention environment as well as to the impact of indefinite detention on family and peer relationships [29]. The disruption of children's attachment relationships, with separation of family groups (usually the removal of fathers), was noted to be particularly traumatizing to already vulnerable children and was associated with attachment disorders. Clinicians described several patterns of disturbed attachment behavior in detained children, including social withdrawal, socially indiscriminate behaviors, and role reversal in relationships with children caring for distressed parents. A number of inquiries noted the inadequate nature of health and mental health services available, particularly for children and adolescents. The 2004 HREOC inquiry reported endemic self-harm and suicidal behavior among young people and the use of isolation and observation as the sole way of responding to this situation by detention authorities. A broader question has been raised about the suitability of the detention environment for the treatment of mental health problems when the regimen and environment themselves are seen as major contributors to the high rates of distress [30]. The medical and mental health bodies united in lobbying the government for the release of children and unaccompanied minors from detention and the placement of detainees who had mental health issues in appropriate treatment [29,31].

An investigation into false detention of an Australian citizen suffering from schizophrenia and the failure of detention staff to recognize or respond to her psychosis highlighted the issue of mental health in detainee populations [32]. There has been a concession on the part of governing bodies that prolonged detention is related to increasing rates of mental health issues; this acknowledgment has been accompanied by a move to treat asylum seekers and detainees who have mental illnesses or mental disorders in either community detention or mental health facilities, as indicated by clinical needs. The provision of mental health services to detention facilities has been increased, and an independent expert advisory group of health professionals including psychiatrists and psychologists (the Detention Expert Health Advisory Group), with a standing mental health subcommittee, has been established. This group is undertaking reviews of mental health and psychosocial screening and assessment protocols and the management of self-harm and suicidal behavior in detention centers. Following a series of highly publicized cases of wrongful detention and mismanagement in 2006 [32], all children and families have been housed in community detention facilities with the support of nongovernment agencies such as the Red Cross. Although this scheme has not been evaluated formally, a significant concern is the lack of access to specialist mental health services for trauma and torture survivors and the lack of expertise with these populations among mainstream mental health services.

Psychological impact of detention on children

As indicated previously, the bulk of evidence regarding the psychological impact of detention on children has emerged from inquiries and research undertaken into the operation of the mandatory detention policy in Australia. Data from a variety of sources, including several Commissions of Inquiry evaluating detention centers and observations of health professionals working in the centers, raise serious concerns about the negative effect of detention on child development and mental health. Limited systematic research also finds that detention per se is a risk factor for the development of mental disorder in children. These findings are summarized in the following sections.

Commissions of inquiry

Several inquiries conducted by the Australian government and by statutory bodies and external inquiries such as that conducted by the United Nation have been reported between 1992 and 2005. A number of the Commissions raised concerns that children's mental health has been affected negatively by their experiences in immigration detention centers. The inquiries have found that these environments compromise parents' abilities to protect their children and to parent effectively. Significantly, the experience of detention itself emerges as an independent and clear risk factor for the development of mental disorder. The conditions of detention, including poor facilities and health services and exposure of children to violence and trauma, have been criticized repeatedly [15].

Depression has been the most common mental disorder described in detainee populations and seems to become more severe with increasing length of time in detention [33,34]. Several Commissions of Inquiry noted that detainees developed depressed mood with associated physical complaints and suicidal ideation and behaviors [28,35]. Self-harm and depression also was noted in children and adolescents, with mass outbreaks of self-harm among adolescents. In 2004 the Department of Human Services, South Australia reported

> Since January 2002, a total of 50 reports of self-harm have been raised on 22 children, ranging in age from 7 to 17 years of age. These incidents included hanging attempts, self-harm by cutting arms or ingesting shampoo; and persistent depression and/or suicidal thoughts. The most frequent incidents occurred with children who are 10–12 years of age. Children aged 14 years are the next highest sub-category represented in this group .... Sixty percent of these reports related to children aged 12 years or less (p. 410) [24].

There was a case report of serious suicidal behavior in a prepubertal girl resulting in prolonged psychiatric hospitalization. Prolonged detention was seen to be related to progressive mental deterioration, hopelessness, and suicidal behavior. The 1998 HREOC inquiry stated

> The human cost is apparent in the evidence of mental distress such as depression, boredom, sleeplessness, psychotic episodes, self harm and suicide attempts. ...The evidence suggests that the indeterminacy of detention makes detention considerably more difficult to endure (p. 218) [28].

The Commonwealth Ombudsman 20001 stated

> While I recognize that detention periods can be extended when refused applicants enter the appeals process, it is clear that long-term detention of immigration detainees is a source of frustration, despondency and depression often resulting in drastic action being taken by the detainees. This I note has been manifested in many recorded incidents of self-harm, hunger strikes and attempted suicide (p. 20) [35].

The 2004 HREOC inquiry into the detention of child asylum seekers in Australia heard from expert witnesses that child development and mental health were affected negatively by inadequate educational facilities, lack of stimulation, and inadequate opportunities for play and peer interaction. In addition, parents themselves frequently were depressed and unable to protect children or to be emotionally available and interactive. Families also were subject to separation, usually of fathers from women and children. The report states:

> The evidence before the inquiry clearly demonstrates that detention centers can have a serious and detrimental impact on the mental health of children. A variety of factors contribute to mental health problems for children in detention. All of them are either the direct result of, or exacerbated by, long-term detention in Australia's detention centers. The longer children are in detention the more likely they will suffer mental harm (p. 429) [24].

Observations were made of children exhibiting socially indiscriminate behaviors and some being in role-reversed relationships with depressed and poorly functioning parents. Clinicians described young children with global developmental delay related to the lack of interaction and stimulation.

A psychologist from the remote Woomera detention facility gave evidence to the 2004 HREOC inquiry that he

> saw parents daily in detention as a result of the stress of detention. Over time, many lost their ability to function effectively as parents and I saw family relationships break down. Parents felt guilty for what they thought they had done to their family in bringing them into this environment (p. 375) [24].

Young children were noted to be particularly vulnerable both to the impact of detention on their parents and to the traumatizing environment itself. Clinicians described children with symptoms of anxiety and disturbed attachment behaviors and emotional regression evidenced by incontinence and sleep disturbance. A child psychiatrist commented that

> children who are in the center for long periods manifest a significant regression over the period of detention. In my opinion, many factors contribute to this regression, over and above the issues within individual families. These factors include: cognitively impoverished conditions, with little opportunity for play and legitimate academic pursuits; reduced availability (physical and emotional) of attachment figures: interference with normal family rituals of feeding and caring; lack of privacy; hostile and deprived physical environment with intimidating and ever-present security measures; dehumanizing use of numbers rather than names; and exposure to violence (not only witnessing full scale riots, but also equally disturbing episodes such as men burying themselves and inviting family to sit around and watch them die). It is hard to conceive of an environment more potentially toxic to child development (p. 397) [24].

Research

Although difficult to conduct, some initial observational research in the Australian context highlighted concerns. In 2001 and 2002 a team of child psychiatrists conducted observations of children held in a remote facility and noted a range of significant emotional disturbances in detained children and adolescents [36] including depression, behavioral dysregulation, and enuresis, with many families being forced to dry children's mattresses in the sun during the day. Two adolescents displayed marked depression and traumatic preoccupation concerning both their premigration experience and experiences in the detention environment. Sultan and O'Sullivan [33] noted that symptoms of separation anxiety, disruptive conduct, nocturnal enuresis, sleep disturbance, and impaired cognitive development were common among children held at one detention facility. At the most severe end of the spectrum, the authors noted that a number of children displayed profound symptoms of psychological distress, including mutism, stereotypic behaviors, and refusal to eat or drink. The authors detailed a pattern of progressive deterioration across the course of detention with marked emotional and behavioral disturbance beginning to emerge after the 6-month period, particularly once initial applications for refugee protection had failed.

Steel and colleagues [37] reported on the findings of structured telephone assessments undertaken in a sample of 10 families detained for 2 to 3 years. The Schedule for Affective Disorders and Schizophrenia for School-Age Children (K-SADS-PL) was administered separately to children and their parents by a team of same-language psychologists. Adult mental disorder was assessed using the Structured Clinical Interview for *Diagnostic and Statistical Manual for Mental Disorders*, (SCID-IV). All parents met criteria for major depressive disorder, and the majority also had posttraumatic stress disorder (PTSD). One third had made suicide attempts while in detention, many in the presence of their children because of the confined nature of the detention environment. The 20 children assessed showed similar signs of distress; all met diagnostic criteria for at least one psychiatric disorder, including major depression, PTSD, separation anxiety disorder, enuresis, and oppositional defiant disorder. About half the children described suicidal ideation, and a quarter had engaged in self-harming behavior. The authors reported that the predetention symptom levels (using the lifetime module of the K-SADS-PL) suggested low levels of psychiatric disturbance before arrival in Australia.

A second investigation of families in detention was reported by Mares and Jureidini [38], who provided psychiatric services for a 2-year period in one of the remote facilities in Australia. The authors report on psychiatric assessments of 16 adults and 20 children age 11 months to 28 years. Diagnosis was based on a series of detailed clinical interviews, undertaken by a range of experienced mental health clinicians over time, to develop consensus diagnoses on each individual child and adult assessed. All the 10 children aged 5 years displayed a cognitive delay. All children aged 7 to 17 years fulfilled criteria for PTSD and major depression with suicidal ideation. All these children described intrusive, disturbing images of trauma experienced in detention. The authors also noted that the mental state of the children and families assessed deteriorated during the treatment period.

These studies clearly suggest that prolonged detention and the exposure of children to trauma in detention combines with the impairment of parental support to produce significant risks for child mental health. The studies and reports undertaken with detained children have a number of important limitations. All are limited by small sample sizes reflecting the difficulty of gaining access to these environments. The research by Mares and Jureidini related to a treated population, although the authors estimate that their sample represented half of the families in that facility with similar clinical reports but not seen by the Child and Adolescent Mental Health Services. The possibility of transcultural error must be acknowledged, but findings using quite different methodologies are consistent. For instance, although Steel and colleagues' [37] study was potentially limited by reliance on a cross-sectional design, Mares and Jureidini [38] documented similar findings using prospective assessments. Similarly, remarkably consistent diagnostic outcomes were identified using both service-based clinical assessments [38] and structured diagnostic interviews [37]. These findings also are consistent with the findings of a larger survey of 200 Vietnamese children held in closed detention in Hong Kong in the early 1990s. McCallin [39] reports that the majority of children presented with symptoms of depression and anxiety, that 52% of those who had high levels of stress had experienced threats to their safety while in detention, and 50% experienced threats during their flight. The study concludes that trauma experienced in detention, including exposure to riots and violence, acted in a cumulative way with feelings of isolation and loss to produce high levels of psychological disturbance.

Vulnerability and risk factors in child asylum seekers—issues of psychological and developmental concern

Children and exposure to trauma in detention

Among asylum seekers, children are particularly vulnerable to the effects of both premigration trauma and their experiences in seeking asylum. The capacity of children to cope with the asylum-seeking experience is complex and depends on the severity of premigration experiences, the child's developmental stage, and the responses of adult caretakers. The predicament of the asylum-seeking child is compounded by the high rates of trauma and distress in parents who essentially are emotionally unavailable for the child. In other traumatized populations it has been observed that rates of PTSD in children can be predicted largely by rates of PTSD in parents, suggesting that parents have a crucial role in promoting trauma adaptation in their children and may serve as a buffer protecting children in the face of traumatic experiences [40,41]. Children in detention witness the breakdown of behavioral control, adult distress and protest behavior, and suicide attempts and self-harm; in some centers, these responses may occur on a mass scale. Children's drawings of these events tend to suggest that they are experiencing overwhelming trauma with no sense of adult protection. The pictures depict scenes of riots and violence and injured detainees. The figures in the drawings are isolated and unprotected, and many have no facial features. The drawings uniformly show the barbed wire fences and razor wire. Older children and adolescents may participate in protests and are acutely aware of the injustice of their situation. This awareness of injustice might affect later social adjustment to the host country.

Parenting in detention

In the detention center environment, parenting as a means of providing care and protection is fundamentally compromised. Parents are essentially unable to provide children with a secure base experience. Parents interviewed in detention describe feelings of guilt and shame and experience a sense of failure in the parental role [24]. Cases have come to light in which parents have attempted suicide in the hope that their children will be released [24]. In the face of indefinite detention, parents may lose hope, and depression contributes to their withdrawal from their children. Observations of children in detention environments suggest that rates of attachment disorder and indiscriminate attachment are high, reflecting parental unavailability.

In the Australian context, the needs of women during pregnancy and delivery and the impact of detention on perinatal mental health also have been raised. Clinicians report that women have been unable to deliver their children according to cultural traditions with appropriate support persons and that in some cases they have been isolated for several weeks before delivery. The lack of interpreters has contributed to fear and distress in complicated deliveries. Clinical evidence suggests that these negative experiences around delivery contribute to the high observed rates of postnatal depression and anxiety as well as to attachment difficulties with infants.

Women asylum seekers are likely to have particular health and mental health needs related to pregnancy and delivery, exacerbated by limited antenatal medical care or screening. Of particular concern are women who have experienced sexual assault and abuse; those whose infants are the products of rape; those who have a history of pregnancy loss, neonatal loss, or early infant death; and first-time mothers in the absence of cultural support. A significant issue in some populations may be genital mutilation, which may also require expert gynecologic and obstetric attention.

Little research is available on pregnant women, but the experience in the United Kingdom seems comparable to that of Australian clinicians. Mcleish and colleagues [42] report on a qualitative interview-based study on a convenience sample of four pregnant and postnatal women in detention facilities in the United Kingdom. The United Kingdom Immigration Services has stated that pregnant women should be detained only in very exceptional circumstances and for brief periods, when no alternatives are possible. The interviewed women had been detained for periods of several months and had high expressed levels of distress, physical discomfort, and concerns about their baby's growth and development. The women described inconsistent antenatal care, including routine screens and investigation, lack of experience in center medical staff, and concerns about the nutritional suitability of the available food for pregnant women. The women with infants had concerns about the availability of infant food and care, and all women described a sense of isolation and lack of competence in the parenting role. They felt guilty and ashamed that they had delivered an infant in detention and were concerned that the infant would be psychologically harmed. The investigators conclude that

The use of prolonged detention for pregnant women and mothers with young children inflicts physical and psychological harm disproportionate to the policy aim of immigration control and should be stopped immediately [42].

Case example: Maya

Maya was a pregnant 26-year-old woman when she was detained in a remote center in Australia following her flight from a Middle Eastern state. She had witnessed the execution of her father and brothers before escaping and was forced to separate from her mother. She was pregnant with her first child and had minimal antenatal care. At 7 months' gestation she was suffering from anxiety and depressive symptoms and was eating poorly. On clinical examination the infant was reported to be small for gestational date. Maya had difficulty eating and was underweight. At 8 months' gestation she was placed in a motel room near the hospital in the town closest to the detention center. She remained under guard but had no available interpreter. She had a complicated delivery and did not understand what was happening to her. She had no support person with her during the delivery. After delivery, she was returned with her baby to the detention facility. She developed an episiotomy-site infection and a urinary tract infection, which were not treated until a delayed check at 6 weeks. She felt anxious and progressively more depressed and isolated herself from her husband, who was placed separately in another section of the detention center. She ruminated on the fate of her baby and considered killing herself and the baby. Twelve months after delivery Maya and her husband were transferred with their baby to a city detention facility. There, a psychiatric consultation found her to be significantly depressed. She was withdrawn, not eating to the extent that she was dehydrated, and suicidal. She complained of breast pain and was found to have bilateral mastitis. Ongoing pelvic pain and discharge was found to be caused by untreated infection. The infant was failing to thrive, emotionally neglected, and globally developmentally delayed. The father was severely depressed and guilty. Both parents required urgent hospitalization and treatment for depression.

Separated children

Children and adolescents are particularly vulnerable during war and conflict. Significant numbers are separated from parents or adult caregivers or are orphaned. Children may be in situations in which they head households and care for younger siblings. All these situations carry increased risks of exploitation and abuse. Children are targeted deliberately in political and ethnic conflicts and for trafficking in forced labor, child pornography, and prostitution. The use of children as soldiers, with associated abuse, is widespread. These children are entitled to seek asylum and protection in the same manner as adult asylum seekers but will have specific needs and mental health issues.

Accurate data on the numbers of separated children seeking asylum are difficult to obtain [43]. UNHCR statistics indicate that nearly 70,000 separated children applied for asylum in 28 industrialized countries during the 4-year period from 1999 to 2003. Data from the United Kingdom [44] report

6900 applications for asylum from separated children in 2002 and 3180 applications in 2003. Despite the increased vulnerability of children at times of conflict, asylum applications by children are less likely than adult applications to be accepted and are more likely to result in discretionary leave to remain in the United Kingdom until 18 years of age, without full assessment of their right to application under the Refugee Convention [45].

Bhabha and colleagues [43] have undertaken an analysis of the reception and processing of separated children in Australia, the United Kingdom, and the United States. In all three countries, they identified inadequate procedures for distinguishing unaccompanied or separated children from other populations. Reception and initial assistance procedures created significant hurdles at very early stages in the process, when vulnerability and need for adult guidance were greatest. None of the legal systems studied provide any formal advice or briefings for children entering the asylum system, and no adequate guardian-like figure was provided to look after the best interests of the children. This lack is coupled with inadequate or nonexistent legal representation and with a lack of child-specific training of officials that results in inappropriate interviewing techniques and questions, aggressive cross-examination, and an intimidating atmosphere. Another pervasive feature found by the authors was the hostile climate, identified by the authors as a widespread "culture of disbelief," that undermines children's confidence in the proceedings.

Child-specific forms of persecution, such as domestic slavery, trafficking, forced marriage, female genital mutilation, and abuse of street children, may be underrecognized and not fully assessed. Children also may underreport the use of torture by state authorities and fail to report inhuman and degrading treatment. Family tracing is also problematic, in that children are likely to be reluctant to provide information regarding family members or their whereabouts. Young children, in particular, may experience feelings of self-blame regarding the fate of family members or believe that they should be rescuing those left behind.

Case example: Eli

Eli, age 7 years, was referred for psychiatric assessment by a nongovernment agency coordinating his care and protection in the community. He had arrived from Central Africa 6 months previously and had been separated from his family for the past 2 years. It was thought that his mother and father had been murdered and that Eli was separated from his two older brothers. He was located in a refugee camp and was cared for by a man from his own community. Eli was resettled in Australia, but his caregiver was denied permission to accompany him. Eli had been placed in a foster placement with a family who also were refugees from Central Africa. He presented with marked withdrawal and depression and was reluctant to eat or drink. He cried constantly and would not describe any experiences before his arrival at the camp. He would say only that, when he was 16 years old, he would return to Africa and look for his brothers whom he had lost. He admitted to having nightmares and at school was described as inattentive and unfocussed.

Emergence of severe psychiatric conditions in asylum-seeking children

A particularly vulnerable population may be children developing a severe life-threatening withdrawal syndrome, as described recently in the Swedish clinical literature. In a group of children of asylum-seeking families, clinicians have observed a presentation thought to be a reaction to extreme stress in association with particular family dynamics and feelings of hopelessness and helplessness. Children become increasingly withdrawn and enter a state of "depressive devitalization" [46]. This syndrome seems comparable to the previously described pervasive refusal syndrome [47–49] occurring in situations of disturbed family relationships.

Clinically the child who has a depressive devitalization syndrome presents with withdrawal, mutism, refusal to eat and drink, and loss of reaction to painful stimuli. The Karolinska Institute describes a series of 16 children, aged 7 to 12 years, presenting between 2002 and 2004 [46]. Fourteen children came from former Soviet republics, and 11 were first-born children. All children had suicidal ideation, and 10 had attempted suicide. Ten mothers had a history of psychiatric treatment for depression, suicidal behaviors, and PTDS. Seven of the families had received negative immigration decisions. All the children were treated as inpatients and required nasogastric feeding. Recovery was noted to commence when the family's immigration status was resolved. A particular feature noted was the mother's symbiotic relationship with the child and the child's positive response to improvement in the mother's mental state.

Although the status of this syndrome remains unclear, it probably is best understood as an extreme reaction to stress in asylum-seeking children when parents are particularly traumatized and unable to exert any moderating effect on the child's experience of the situation. It remains unclear whether any culturally specific factors contribute to this presentation, how generalized it is, or if the Swedish experience is unique. Pre-existing vulnerability seems likely and includes disturbances of the mother–child relationship, maternal psychopathology, and poor stress tolerance.

Advocacy, ethics, and dilemmas for clinicians

Many clinicians involved in work with detained asylum seekers have commented on the inherent difficulties of providing meaningful intervention in this setting. A fundamental dilemma emerges when the nature of the environment itself is seen as contributing in a major way to detainees' mental health issues. For children, this situation is even more acute when their overall development is compromised by environmental neglect and the impact of detention on family functioning. These issues affect the clinical role and raise issues about the effectiveness of clinical interventions.

Case example: SB

The highly publicized case of SB, a 7-year-old boy in detention, highlights clinicians' concerns about the undermining of their clinical role and the need to advocate on behalf of a child patient.

SB initially presented at 6 years of age when he was withdrawn and refusing to talk or drink. He had been in detention with his family for 14 months and while in a remote facility had witnessed acute distress and riots among detainees and mass self-harming behaviors including attempted self-immolation. SB developed features of acute traumatic response with bed-wetting, chronic sleep disturbance, and nightmares. When transferred to another urban detention center, he again witnessed outbreaks of self-harm and was exposed to a severe wrist-cutting episode. He became progressively more withdrawn and mute. On admission to a hospital he was dehydrated but began describing preoccupations with the self-harming behaviors he had witnessed. He was diagnosed as having PTSD, and psychiatric opinions were given that he should not be returned to the detention center, which terrified him, but that he should be released into the community with his primary caregiver. This clinical advice was ignored, and on return to the center SB relapsed, requiring readmission for hydration within 1 week. Hospital staff proposed to the Department of Immigration that detention clearly would result in relapse and was not in the best interests of the child. Clinicians saw their role as one of advocating for and protecting the child, which put them in direct conflict with government. A significant political discussion rapidly embroiled the medical and broader community. SB was readmitted multiple times as the debate continued and remains in treatment several years later, despite being with his family in the community. He has received large financial compensation.

Clinicians' reporting on their experiences in working within remote detention centers described their increasing feelings of powerlessness, anger, and guilt as the limitations of their role became apparent. Many initially had hoped that they were equipped to treat and support traumatized children and adults but felt increasingly impotent in the face of a merciless government policy and the petty tyrannies of a detention environment run along the lines of a penal colony. Numerous reports were made of clinical recommendations being ignored and dismissed as biased or inaccurate in a culture that saw the detainees as simulating distress and engaging in so-called "manipulative behaviors." Clinicians have described their experience of "vicarious traumatization" [50] working with detained children and their parents, with the crucial difference that in this situation the children are in a state of ongoing traumatization or are in fear of the future [51]. Clinicians essentially witnessed the denial of children's human rights and a system that abnegated responsibility for the care and protection of children. Recommendations by child protection workers also made little impact [52].

The awareness of systemic barriers to appropriate care and of the human rights violations made great impact on clinicians, most of whom had not previously confronted political dilemmas of this kind [51,53,54]. This experience forced a review of the boundaries of the clinical role, with some arguing that clinicians have an ethical responsibility to challenge the government when harm is done to individuals and groups as a result of bad law and policy [55,56]. Remaining silent and acting as a bystander in effect colludes with the harmful practices. In Australia a group of medical and health bodies (the Professional Alliance for the Health of Asylum Seekers and Their Children) formed to advocate for the release of children and families into the community and for the abolition of the policy of mandatory detention [29].

Summary

An understanding of and response to the high rates of mental disorder among asylum seekers needs to include an understanding of the circumstances of their flight, past trauma, and current situation. This understanding includes an evaluation of current stressors, such as being held indefinitely in detention, being subject to incomprehensible legal and administrative processes, and having little control over daily life. The experience of being a detainee, with limited ways of communicating one's plight, shapes the expression of distress. Clinicians need to see the distress and symptoms of mental disorder as emerging in the context of the detention environment rather than within a traditional medical model. For children this understanding is even more important, because the use of diagnostic labels without elaboration does not provide an adequate account of the child's difficulties. For example, in the case of SD the dilemma was that he could not recover if he was returned to the place that terrified him, a current environmental factor, not that he suffered from PTSD related only to past traumatic exposure. In detained asylum seekers, medication and standard management approaches to distress are unlikely to be effective in the context of ongoing detention and retraumatization. The challenge for clinicians is to acknowledge that the distress experienced by asylum seekers may not be disproportionate to the environmental circumstances in which they find themselves and to accept that treating isolated symptoms is unlikely to be helpful. Clinicians seeing asylum-seeking children have a responsibility to act as advocates for their care and protection and to act at all times in the best interests of the child. Doing so may bring them into conflict with detention center authorities and government policy.

In the face of systems of detention that are damaging, the clinician has an important role in bearing witness to the harm done to detainees as well as trying to prevent harm in whatever way possible. Maintaining clinical records and documenting the impact of detention on mental state over time is vital and should include descriptions of the environmental factors contributing to mental disorder and distress. Diagnosis in this environment needs to be based on broad assessment and history and put in the context of the asylum-seeking experience.

Asylum-seeking children may be one of the most vulnerable groups of displaced persons. Although the clinical role may be undermined by systems of deterrence and inappropriate detention, clinicians have become advocates for the welfare of children and should continue to articulate clearly the ethical principles on which all health practice is based—to prevent what harm they can and to document what they cannot prevent.

References

[1] Kushner T, Knox C. Refugees in an age of genocide. London: Frank Cass; 1999.

[2] Diallo K, Chabaké TA, editors. Statistical yearbook 2005: trends in displacement, protection and solutions. Geneva (Switzerland): United Nations High Commissioner for Refugees; 2007.

[3] United Nations High Commissioner for Refugees. The state of the worlds refugees: in search of solutions. New York: Oxford University Press; 1995.

[4] United Nations High Commissioner for Refugees. State of world's refugees: human displacement in the new millennium. Oxford (UK); 2006.

[5] Silove D, Steel Z, Watters C. Policies of deterrence and the mental health of asylum seekers in Western Countries. JAMA 2000;284:604–11.

[6] Malloch MS, Stanley E. The detention of asylum seekers in the UK—representing risk, managing the dangerous. Punishment & Society-International Journal of Penology 2005;7(1): 53–71.

[7] Klocker N, Dunn KM. Who's driving the asylum debate? Newspaper and government representations of asylum seekers. Media International Australia Incorporating Culture and Policy 2003;109:71–92.

[8] Wilkinson R. Everyone wants to help children. So why are so many millions still suffering? Refugees 2001;122(1):5–7.

[9] United Nations High Commissioner for Refugees. Trends in unaccompanied and separated children seeking asylum in industrialized countries, 2001–2003. Geneva (Switzerland): United Nations High Commissioner for Refugees; 2004.

[10] Silove D, Sinnerbrink I, Field A, et al. Anxiety, depression and PTSD in asylum seekers: associations with pre-migration trauma and post-migration stressors. Br J Psychiatry 1997; 170:351–7.

[11] Silove D, Steel Z, Susljik I, et al. Torture, mental health status and the outcomes of refugee applications among recently arrived asylum seekers in Australia. International Journal of Migration, Health and Social Care 2006;2(1):4–14.

[12] Laban CJ, Gernaat HBPE, Komproe IH, et al. Postmigration living problems and common psychiatric disorders in Iraqi asylum seekers in the Netherlands. J Nerv Ment Dis 2005; 193(12):825–32.

[13] Steel Z, Silove D, Bird K, et al. Pathways from war trauma to posttraumatic stress symptoms among Tamil asylum seekers, refugees, and immigrants. J Trauma Stress 1999; 12(3):421–35.

[14] Iredale R, Mitchell C, Pe-Pua R, et al. Ambivalent welcome: the settlement experiences of humanitarian entrant families in Australia. Wollongong (Australia): NSW Centre for Multicultural Studies; 1996.

[15] Silove D, Austin P, Steel Z. No refuge from terror: the impact of detention on the mental health of trauma-affected refugees seeking asylum in Australia. Transcult Psychiatry 2007; 44(3):359–93.

[16] Women' Commission for Refugee Women and Children. Locking up family values: the detention of immigrant families. 2007. Available at: http://www.womenscommission.org/pdf/famdeten.pdf. Accessed January 14, 2008.

[17] Amnesty International. Italy: temporary stay—permanent rights: the treatment of foreign nationals detained in 'temporary stay and assistance centres' (CPTAs). Italy (Germany): Amnesty International; 2005.

[18] International Detention Coalition. Children in immigration detention position paper. 2007. Available at: http://idcoalition.org/portal/component/option,com_remository/Itemid,105/func,fileinfo/id,161/. Accessed January 14, 2008.

[19] Home Office. Control of immigration: statistics United Kingdom 2006; 2007. Report No.: CM 7197.

[20] Home Office. Control of immigration: statistics United Kingdom 2005; 2006. Report No.: CM 6904.

[21] Immigration and Naturalization Service Office of Juvenile Affairs. Fact sheet. 2002. Available at: http://www.ilw.com/immigdaily/News/2002,0813-juveniles.pdf. Accessed January 14, 2008.

[22] Bhabha J, Schmidt S. Seeking asylum alone: unaccompanied and separated children and refugee protection in the U.S. John D. and Catherine T. MacArthur Foundation. Sydney, Australia: Federation Press; 2006.

[23] US Immigration and Customs Enforcement. The ICE T. Don Hutto Family Residential Facility: maintaining family unity, enforcing immigration laws. 2007. Available at: http://www.ice.gov/pi/news/factsheets/huttofactsheet.htm. Accessed January 14, 2008.

[24] Human Rights and Equal Opportunity Commission. A last resort? National inquiry into children in immigration detention. Sydney (Australia): Human Rights and Equal Opportunity Commmission; 2004.

[25] Dudley M. Contradictory Australian national policies on self-harm and suicide: the case of asylum seekers in mandatory detention. Australas Psychiatry 2003;11(Suppl):s102–8.

[26] Becker R, Silove D. Psychological and psychosocial effects of prolonged detention. In: Crock M, editor. Protection or punishment: the detention of asylum-seekers in Australia. Sydney (Australia): The Federation Press; 1993. p. 81–91.

[27] Silove D, McIntosh P, Becker R. Risk of retraumatisation of asylum-seekers in Australia. Aust N Z J Psychiatry 1993;27(4):606–12.

[28] Human Rights and Equal Opportunity Commission. Those who've come across the seas: the report of the Commission's inquiry into the detention of unauthorised arrivals. Canberra (Australia): Commonwealth of Australia; 1998.

[29] Professional Alliance for the Health of Asylum Seekers and Their Children. Submission to the national inquiry into children in immigration detention. 2002. Available at: http://www.hreoc.gov.au/human_rights/children_detention/submissions/index.html. Accessed January 14, 2008.

[30] McLoughlin PJ. Serve, subvert or emancipate? Promoting mental health in immigration detention. Australian eJouranl for the Advancement of Mental Health 2006;5:1–10.

[31] Australian Medical Association. Media release: asylum seekers should have access to quality health services under Medicare 8 August 2001. Available at: http://www.ama.com.au/web.nsf/doc/WEEN-5GB46R. Accessed April 1, 2008.

[32] Palmer MJ. Inquiry into the circumstances of the immigration detention of Cornelia Rau: report. Canberra (Australia): Commonwealth of Australia; 2005.

[33] Sultan A, O'Sullivan K. Psychological disturbances in asylum seekers held in long term detention: a participant-observer account. Med J Aust 2001;175:593–6.

[34] Steel Z, Silove D, Brooks R, et al. Impact of immigration detention and temporary protection on the mental health of refugees. Br J Psychiatry 2006;188:58–64.

[35] Commonwealth Ombudsman. Report of an own motion investigation into the Department of Immigration and Multicultural Affairs' immigration detention centres. Canberra (Australia): Commonwealth of Australia; 2001.

[36] Mares S, Newman L, Dudley M, et al. Seeking refuge, losing hope: parents and children in immigration detention. Australas Psychiatry 2002;10:91–6.

[37] Steel Z, Momartin S, Bateman C, et al. Psychiatric status of asylum seeker families held for a protracted period in a remote detention centre in Australia. Aust N Z J Public Health 2004; 28(6):527–36.

[38] Mares S, Jureidini J. Psychiatric assessment of children and families in immigration detention: clinical, administrative and ethical issues. Aust N Z J Public Health 2004;28(6):16–22.

[39] McCallin M. Living in detention: a review of the psychological wellbeing of Vietnamese children in the Hong Kong detention centres. Geneva (Switzerland): International Catholic Child Bureau; 1992.

[40] Qouta S, Punamaki RL, Elsavraj E. Mother-child expression of psychological distress in war trauma. Clinical Child Psychiatry and Psychology 2005;10:135–56.

[41] Laon N, Wolmer L, Cohen DJ. Mother's functioning and children's symptoms. Five years after SCUD missile attack. American Journal of Psychiatry 2001;158:1020–6.

[42] Mcleish J, Cutler S, Stancer C. A crying shame: pregnant asylum seekers and their babies in detention. 2002. Available at: http://www.asylumsupport.info/babiesandacryingshame.htm. Accessed January 14, 2008.

[43] Bhabha J, Crock M, Finch N, et al. Seeking asylum alone: unaccompanied and separated children and refugee protection in Australia, the U.K. and the U.S. Sydney (Australia): Federation Press; 2006.

[44] Finch N. Seeking asylum alone. In: Anderson H, Ascher H, Bjornberg U, et al, editors. The asylum-seeking child in Europe. Goteborg (Sweden): Goteborg University; 2005. p. 57–66.

[45] Halvarsen K. Decisions on separated children who apply for asylum. In: Anderson H, Ascher H, Bjornberg U, et al, editors. The asylum-seeking child in Europe. Goteborg (Sweden): Goteborg University; 2005. p. 67–73.

[46] Bodegård G. Pervasive loss of function in asylum-seeking children in Sweden. Acta Paediatr 2005;94:1706–7.

[47] Lask B. Pervasive refusal syndrome. Advances in Psychiatric Treatment 2004;10:153–9.

[48] Lask B, Britten C, Kroll L, et al. Children with pervasive refusal. Arch Dis Child 1991;66: 866–9.

[49] Nunn K, Thompson S. The pervasive refusal syndrome: learned helplessness and hopelessness. Clin Child Psychol Psychiatry 1996;1:121–32.

[50] McCann LI. Vicarious traumatization: a framework for understanding the psychological effects of working with victims. J Trauma Stress 1990;3:131–49.

[51] Steel Z, Mares S, Newman L, et al. The politics of asylum and immigration detention: advocacy, ethics and the professional role of the therapist. In: Wilson J, Drozdek B, editors. Broken spirits: the treatment of traumatized asylum seekers, refugees, war and torture survivors. New York: Brunner-Routledge; 2004. p. 659–87.

[52] Layton R. Best investment: a state plan to protect in advance the interests of children. Child Protection Review 2003;22:14.

[53] Koopowitz LF, Abhary S. Psychiatric aspects of detention: illustrative case studies. Aust N Z J Psychiatry 2004;38(7):495–500.

[54] Koutroulis G. Detained asylum seekers, health care, and questions of human(e)ness. Aust N Z J Public Health 2003;27(4):381–4.

[55] Steel Z, Silove D. Science and the common good: indefinite, non-reviewable mandatory detention of asylum seekers and the research imperative. Monash Bioeth Rev 2004;23(4): 93–103.

[56] McNeill PM. Public health ethics: asylum seekers and the case for political action. Bioethics 2003;17(5–6):487–501.

ELSEVIER
SAUNDERS

Child Adolesc Psychiatric Clin N Am
17 (2008) 685–702

CHILD AND
ADOLESCENT
PSYCHIATRIC CLINICS
OF NORTH AMERICA

The Traumatic Impact of Hurricane Katrina on Children in New Orleans

Stacy S. Drury, MD, PhD*,
Michael S. Scheeringa, MD, MPH,
Charles H. Zeanah, MD

*Department of Psychiatry and Neurology, Tulane University School of Medicine, Health
Science Center, 1440 Canal Street, TB 52, New Orleans, LA 70112, USA*

It is well known that environmental disasters are associated with an increased prevalence of psychiatric disorders [1], and there is some evidence that children may be disproportionately affected [2]. Most environmental disasters involve complex traumas, and the degree of later psychologic disturbance generally is related to the degree of exposure. This article reviews the traumatic impact of Hurricane Katrina on the children of New Orleans. After describing the events comprising the trauma, it reviews the historical context of hurricanes in New Orleans and the social and political challenges that affected the area's response. It then considers the consequences of Hurricane Katrina in terms of disruption of services and governmental and nongovernmental responses to the psychologic needs created by the storm. The authors review preliminary studies about the affects of the hurricane on children and adolescents, and conclude with a consideration of the lessons learned from both practice and policy perspectives.

Background

On August 29, 2005, Hurricane Katrina, one of the worst environmental disasters ever to occur in the United States, struck the Gulf Coast with winds exceeding 125 miles per hour and extending outward for more than 120 miles. More than 90,000 square miles of land were impacted by the storm, and more than 80% of New Orleans flooded following multiple breaches in the levee protection system. It is estimated that more than

---

* Corresponding author. 1440 Canal St TB 52, New Orleans, LA 70112.
E-mail address: sdrury@tulane.edu (S.S. Drury).

1056-4993/08/$ - see front matter © 2008 Elsevier Inc. All rights reserved.
doi:10.1016/j.chc.2008.02.005
childpsych.theclinics.com

5.8 million people lived in the Gulf Coast areas impacted by Hurricane Katrina, of these, 1.5 million lived in the New Orleans metropolitan area. After the storm made landfall, it is estimated that more than 90% of the population of southeast Louisiana evacuated and relocated for weeks to months.

Unlike other environmental disasters, the hurricane itself was followed by a unique succession of events that posed challenges for recovery. Early on, two major breaches of the flood protection walls in the metropolitan area occurred, soon followed by more breaches. Massive and unprecedented flooding was a second major traumatic event for those who remained in New Orleans. Many of those who had evacuated witnessed these events unfolding on television and were filled with uncertainty and dread for friends, families, and their own homes. Following the flooding, a third source of trauma developed—widespread civil unrest characterized by panicked searches for food and water, looting, and violent activity on the streets. Media reports and rumors of violence were more widespread than actual violence, particularly in the "shelters of last resort," the Superdome and the Convention Center. Further, for many reasons, local, state, and federal government responses to these first three sources of trauma were uncoordinated and ineffective, leaving people trapped in various unsafe environments for days, adding abandonment and continuing exposure to danger as additional sources of trauma [3].

Affected population

Estimates from a variety of sources are that 80,000 to 90,000 people remained in New Orleans during the hurricane and that more than 25,000 people were located at the Louisiana Superdome. Using 2000 census data and recorded estimates of individuals at the Superdome and Convention Center, it has been estimated that more than 11,000 children were located at those facilities at some time. In addition, it is estimated that more than 9000 individuals, including 400 children and adolescents, were rescued from flooded homes [3,4].

After the hurricane and subsequent flooding of the city, adults and children who were rescued were taken from New Orleans to sites around the country without planning or documentation, often being separated from their families and with with no clear method for remaining in contact. An unprecedented American diaspora led to residents seeking shelter in all 50 states and a number of foreign countries. The Red Cross initially reported that more than 374,000 people were in shelters, hotels, or alternative homes in the first week after Katrina, but this number increased to more than 1 million as more individuals were able to register with the Red Cross. Estimates of the number of children evacuated and relocated, either temporarily or permanently, range between 200,000 and 370,000 [5,6].

Although many children remained with their families, more than 5192 children were reported missing to the National Center for Missing and

Exploited Children. As late as October, 2005, 2500 children were still missing, and the last of them were not reunited with their families until March 17, 2006 [7]. Estimates from initial screening surveys indicate that one third of children were separated from their primary caregivers at some point during the hurricane, and 10% remained separated 4 to 8 months later [7,8], sometimes because of temporary parental employment needs.

In summary, the citizens of New Orleans and surrounding areas experienced a series of successive traumas: (1) hurricane-force winds causing widespread damage to property and disrupting power and communications; (2) flooding of 80% of the city resulting in increased fatalities, property destruction, and infrastructure collapse; (3) widespread civil unrest in which criminal activity often was unchallenged by an overwhelmed police force; (4) tens of thousands of trapped and abandoned citizens who were not rescued for days; (5) prolonged displacement of nearly 1.5 million people; and (6) separation from family, friends, and social support networks.

Historical context

Several previous hurricanes have struck the Gulf Coast region during the last 50 years, including Hurricane Betsy in 1965 (a category 3 hurricane that struck New Orleans), Hurricane Camille in 1969 (a category 5 hurricane that hit Gulfport, Mississippi), and Hurricane Lili in 2002 (a category 2 hurricane that hit the Intracoastal City of Louisiana). Hurricane Betsy, with winds of 110 miles per hour when it hit New Orleans, resulted in significant flooding of more than 165,000 homes in many areas in greater New Orleans, including the Lower and Upper Ninth Wards, as well as St. Bernard Parish (adjacent to New Orleans). It took more than 10 days for the water to recede after this hurricane. As a result of the failure of the levee system to protect New Orleans, the federal government enacted the Louisiana Hurricane Protection Act.

Congress authorized the construction of a series of levees and concrete walls to protect the areas around Lake Pontchartrain and New Orleans in the "Lake Pontchartrain and Vicinity, Louisiana Hurricane Protection Project" funded through the Flood Control Act of 1965. The initial project, a joint federal, state, and local effort, was anticipated to take 13 years to complete and to cost an estimated $85 million dollars. The plan was to create a system that could protect coastal Louisiana from a category 3 hurricane, which was estimated to occur only about once in every hundred years. During the course of its completion, multiple changes were made to the initial plan, and the cost grew to more than $757 million dollars with an estimated completion date of 2008.

When Hurricane Katrina hit New Orleans, the levee system was 60% to 90% complete. All the breaches in the system occurred in areas that were assumed to have been completed and to be able to withstand the impact of a category 3 hurricane [9]. According to the Army Corps of Engineers, there were concerns even before Hurricane Katrina that the completed flood protection system would not protect New Orleans from a hurricane stronger than category 3, but efforts to evaluate this possibility were just underway when Katrina made landfall.

The impact of Hurricane Katrina also was accentuated by the social and political challenges facing Louisiana, and in particular New Orleans, before the storm. Louisiana, before Katrina, had one of the highest poverty and uninsured rates in the nation, in addition to one of the worst health indicator scores [10]. Evacuation efforts were complicated by tens of thousands of poor people with disabling health problems and a significant proportion of the population without access to transportation. Although a mandatory evacuation order was issued the day before Katrina made landfall, the city's plan to assist in the evacuation of the poor or disabled was not enacted initially and then could not be enacted after the buses and routes of transportation were flooded [11–13]. Despite these problems, more than 90% of the population evacuated before the storm—the most successful evacuation of a large metropolitan area in history.

Consequences of hurricane katrina

Disruption of mental health services

In the initial aftermath of Hurricane Katrina, all nine general hospitals in the city were closed; services remained only in adjacent parishes. A large percentage of the New Orleans metropolitan area, in particular areas that were flooded, did not regain power for weeks to months. Community mental health clinics, which provided nearly all the psychiatric care to the poor and uninsured in Orleans Parish, were closed, leaving patients without medications, medical records, or available care. Child and adolescent inpatients from the New Orleans Adolescent Hospital were evacuated to the state forensic hospital in Jackson, Louisiana, where some remained for months [14].

Considerable attention has been paid in the media to the disruption of services, particularly inpatient services, for chronically mentally ill adults caused by Hurricane Katrina, including loss of mental health professionals [15–18]. In contrast, the traumatic effects of the storm, particularly its impact on children and adolescents, have received much less emphasis, and no comprehensive approach to address the mental health needs of children and adolescents has been instituted.

Governmental responses

Following the Hurricane Katrina disaster, the federal government allocated more than $44 million to Louisiana for disaster mental health response through the procedures established by the Federal Emergency Management Agency (FEMA). In addition, the federal government allocated $220 million in Social Services Block Grant funds to Louisiana in February 2006. Despite these allocations, there has been no coordinated effort to date either to treat affected individuals or to train clinicians in evidence-based approaches for disaster-related mental health disorders. The reasons for this disconnect have implications for responses to future disasters.

The federal emergency management agency and the substance abuse and mental health services administration

In 1974, the United States Congress passed the Robert T. Stafford Disaster Relief and Emergency Assistance Act that formalized mechanisms to access a wide range of federal assistance following emergencies. The mental health response is described as "crisis counseling" and is defined as "professional counseling services, including financial assistance to State or local agencies or private mental health organizations to provide such services or training...." [19].

FEMA has an interagency agreement to manage the mental health component after disasters with the Substance Abuse and Mental Health Services Administration (SAMHSA), which has opted to interpret the Stafford Act to mean that FEMA funds after disasters cannot be used for mental health treatment. A subdivision of SAMHSA, the Emergency Mental Health and Traumatic Stress Services Branch, manages the mental health component, which generally is referred to as the "Crisis Counseling Program" (CCP). The CCP is not mental health treatment and is intended to be short-term (meaning fewer than five sessions). The CCP generally is provided by nonlicensed laypersons; endorsed activities include "providing emotional support, and encouraging linkages with other individuals and agencies who may help." For those who truly need treatment, however, crisis counseling is primarily a referral program.

Unfortunately, there is absolutely no evidence that crisis counseling helps people who do not have substantial mental health needs recover more quickly or more fully, and there is no evidence demonstrating the crisis counseling fulfills its referral function of helping people who do have acute mental health needs—whether produced or exacerbated by the crisis—find treatment providers. There also is no evidence that crisis counseling can "encourage the use of mental health services by reducing discrimination and stigma associated with receiving them." These problems result in part from a requirement, intended to reduce stigma, that all contacts between crisis counselors and individuals be anonymous. Furthermore, no screening instrument is used for systematic assessment of distress. In fact, no formal measures of any kind are required. Thus, despite governmental endorsement, there is limited evidence to support crisis counseling as an effective intervention after disasters at any level.

A report that was created in the aftermath of the 2004 and 2005 hurricanes by the Congressional Research Service, noted, "The actual effect of the program on health outcomes has not been demonstrated" [20]. The report went on to document that in 2002 the Government Accountability Office had "recommended that FEMA and SAMHSA collaborate in evaluating the effectiveness of CCP," noting that the FEMA Inspector General had made the same recommendation in 1995. No evaluation has taken place.

The Louisiana Department of Social Services has used some of its Block Grant funds to support various mental health initiatives. For example, it provided supplemental funding to an ongoing intervention for young maltreated children in foster care [21]. It also supported a program designed by Columbia University and run by the Jefferson Parish Human Services Authority to operate in 35 Jefferson Parish schools [22]. This program, The School Therapeutic Enhancement Program, focuses on depression and disruptive behavior but curiously, not on posttraumatic stress disorder (PTSD).

Nongovernmental responses

Private foundations have provided much of the support for meaningful treatment in the aftermath of Katrina, often through universities and local agencies. The following is a list of selected examples of programs that have been supported.

The Kellogg Foundation provided $12,000,000, the largest single contribution to disaster recovery in the foundation's history [23]. Some of this support is for children's mental health treatment services, especially school-based mental health interventions. Tulane Child and Adolescent Psychiatry is providing school-based services through this program.

The Catholic Archdiocese of New Orleans funded the Fleur de Lis project to provide tiered support and triage in school settings for children who have mental health and learning challenges [24]. Initially, this project was conducted within the parochial school system in greater New Orleans, but it since has expanded into other school systems. By September 2007, the project involved children and teachers from 50 schools in greater New Orleans.

The Institute for Mental Hygiene, a New Orleans focused foundation, provided the largest grant in its history for implementation of a learning supports model of mental health interventions in two new charter schools in New Orleans. This effort is an attempt to develop a model of services, ranging from creating a mentally healthy climate in the classroom, to enhanced classroom support for teachers, to inclusion of integrated mental health services on site when necessary. The goal of the project is to test a model that is coherent but also adaptable to individual schools [25].

Other nonprofit agencies and universities have obtained funding for various targeted efforts. Under the sponsorship of the Children's Health Fund, for example, two mobile children's health clinics that include counseling, therapy, and child psychiatric services currently are providing free services in Orleans and St. Bernard Parish [26]. What continues to be lacking is a comprehensive and coordinated approach to the traumatic experiences that tens of thousands of children and adolescents and their parents suffered during and after Hurricane Katrina. Significant PTSD impairment was predicted in a needs assessment completed 6 weeks after Hurricane Katrina [3], and ongoing research has documented clearly that the predictions about the scope of the need were largely correct.

In essence, two major approaches to the disruption of services caused by Hurricane Katrina have been employed. First, there have been efforts to restore infrastructure and to provide services by working through extant structures that recovered soon after the storm. Although major systems were disrupted, some could be re-established, perhaps configured differently than before the storm [27]. For children, many clinics and even hospitals in parishes outside of the city reopened early and could be used to provide services. In areas of the city that did not flood, clinics reopened and served former residents even if they had relocated temporarily outside of the city. For example, the Orleans Parish Early Childhood Supports and Services clinic reopened in New Orleans and served former residents who had relocated to Jefferson, St. Bernard, and St. Tammany Parishes. (Before Katrina, services were restricted families residing within the city.) A second response has been to develop new programs and services, such as the school-based services noted earlier. What has been missing is an overarching plan for restoring services and for addressing the needs of affected children.

Mental health consequences for children

A survey conducted by the Kaiser Foundation in early 2007 of 1500 randomly selected adults in New Orleans found that 15% of adults rated their mental health as worse after Hurricane Katrina, 4% of parents reported that their children exhibited new behavior problems, and 9% indicated that their children did not get needed health care in the last 6 months [28]. Surveys of adults in the aftermath of Katrina have documented enormous psychiatric morbidity [29,30]. This morbidity has obvious implications for children, because depression, anxiety, PTSD, and substance abuse documented in adults are known to be associated with compromised care giving and increased child psychopathology [31]. Furthermore, some adolescents have returned to the city without parents, living in varying degrees of instability with relatives or acquaintances [32], but their actual numbers are not known.

Studies of children conducted to date, summarized in Table 1, range from brief surveys to well-validated questionnaires to structured psychiatric interviews. Studies reporting child symptomatology include both children and parents. Children in some of the studies had been studied before Katrina, and data about them provide important insights into risks for psychopathology. Results from two interventions also have been published. What is most striking about the results from these studies, despite differences in design and methodology, is that they largely converge on several conclusions.

Table 1
Studies of the effects of Hurricane Katrina and interventions afterwards

Study	Sample	Number in study	Outcome measures	Findings
Effects				
Osofsky, et al (2007) [8]	Parents of children enrolled in head start and a sample of fourth through twelfth graders from Orleans, St. Bernard, and St. John the Baptist Parishes; 48% white, 42% African American; 4% Hispanic; gender not specified	2192 school-age children and parents of 787 children in Head Start through third grade	An interview designed to cover experiences during the hurricane was developed for use in investigation; Children fourth grade and older reported on themselves; parents of younger children reported on their symptoms.	In school-age children, 50% exceeded clinical cutoff; common symptoms were depression, loneliness, sadness, and anger (one third of the respondents). They also reported distress at reminders, anhedonia, and difficulty concentrating. In of younger children 27% exceeded clinical cutoff.
Weems, et al (2007) [37]	School-age children and adolescents (mean age, 11 years) who had participated in studies before Katrina; ethnicity not specified; 58% male	52 children who had been studied before Katrina were assessed after Katrina	Child Posttraumatic Stress Disorder Checklist (Amaya-Jackson et al, 1995)	Symptoms of PTSD and depression were reported; separation anxiety and clinginess were most common. Children had mild-to-moderate PTSD symptomatology. Trait anxiety and negative affect before Katrina were predictors of posttraumatic stress symptoms following the hurricane, even after pre-Katrina posttraumatic symptoms and hurricane-related events were taken into account. Pre-Katrina GAD symptoms predicted postdisaster GAD symptoms, and pre-Katrina trait anxiety predicted post-Katrina depressive symptoms.

Scaramella, et al [36]	Mothers and toddlers enrolled in Head Start	55 mothers and their 24-month-old children recruited before Katrina and 47 mothers and their 24-month-old children recruited after Katrina	Maternal depression assessed by Symptom Checklist-90-Revised (SCL-90-R; Derogatis, 1983). Mothers' parenting effectiveness measured by scale constructed for study. Child Behavior Checklist for ages 2–3 years (Achenbach, 1994).	Financial strain and neighborhood violence were associated with higher levels of depressed mood in mothers; depressed mood was linked to less parenting efficacy. Poor parenting efficacy was associated with more child internalizing and externalizing problems. Exposure to the hurricane did not moderate these relationships, because there were no differences in pre-Katrina and post-Katrina samples.
Hensley and Varela [34]	Students from public and private schools in New Orleans; 46% African American, 37% white; 8% Hispanic, 6% Asian/Pacific Islander; 61% male	302 sixth and seventh graders in New Orleans surveyed 5–8 months after Katrina	Posttraumatic stress symptomatology in children was measured using the Reaction Index for Children format (Frederick et al, 1992). Somatic symptoms were measured with the Children's Somatization Index (Garber et al, 1991).	Hurricane exposure was a significant predictor of PTSD symptoms and somatic symptoms. Also, as hypothesized, anxiety sensitivity differentially moderated the influence of trait anxiety on PTSD symptoms and somatic symptoms. Hurricane exposure and trait anxiety were unique predictors of PTSD symptoms after controlling for gender effects, together accounting for 46% of the variance in PTSD symptoms.

(continued on next page)

Table 1 (*continued*)

Study	Sample	Number in study	Outcome measures	Findings
Scheeringa and Zeanah [35]	Children between the age of 36 and 72 months living in New Orleans at the time of Hurricane Katrina; 56% African American, 31% white; 57% male	70 preschool children recruited from newspaper advertisements; 66% had been evacuated before Katrina, and 34% stayed through Katrina	Psychiatric symptoms, disorders and impairment derived from Preschool Age Psychiatric Assessment (Egger et al, 2006) as reported by mothers; A Disaster Experiences Questionnaire was developed to assess experiences during and after Katrina	Children's rate of PTSD was 50.0% overall (62.5% of those who stayed in the city; 43.5% of those who evacuated before Katrina). Within the group that remained in the city, there were no differences in those who were separated from caregivers and those who were not. For children who had PTSD, 88.6% had at least one comorbid disorder (ODD and SAD were most common). New-onset disorders after Katrina occurred exclusively in children who also developed PTSD following Katrina.
Interventions following Hurricane Katrina				
Weems, et al [33]	Ninth-grade students from New Orleans; Predominantly African American; 44% male	94 students were assessed 13 months after Katrina but before intervention; 73 students were assessed 20 months after Katrina and after the intervention; 30 students completed the intervention.	After screening for exposure to traumatic experiences and distress related to Hurricane Katrina, Test Anxiety and PTSD symptoms at 13 months post-Katrina, a group intervention comprising relaxation training and hierarchical exposures that was designed to reduce test anxiety was administered. Follow-up measures were obtained 20 months after Katrina.	Level of exposure to the hurricane were related to severity of posttraumatic symptoms. The intervention reduced test anxiety and improved academic performance. The intervention also reduced posttraumatic symptoms, and a change in test anxiety was a predictor of change in PTSD symptoms.

| Salloum and Overstreet [38] | Second through sixth grade children; 89% African American; 62.5% male | 56 school-aged children were assigned randomly to individualized intervention or group intervention. | Manualized 10-week intervention using techniques from cognitive behavioral therapy and narrative therapy administered to children in either in individual or group format. | Children in both intervention groups had significant reductions in posttraumatic stress symptoms, depression, traumatic grief, and distress. There was no difference in children who received individual or group interventions. There was a trend for younger girls to have more PTSD symptoms. |

Abbreviations: GAD, generalized anxiety disorder; ODD, oppositional defiant disorder; PTSD, posttraumatic stress disorder; SAD, seasonal affective disorder.

First, Hurricane Katrina and its aftermath clearly have been associated with serious psychopathology in children and adolescents. Toddlers through adolescents have been included in the studies listed in Table 1, and all have demonstrated high levels of disturbance. Although PTSD is best documented, various signs and symptoms of depression, anxiety, disruptive behavior, and somatic complaints have been identified [33–38]. As one example, Scheeringa and Zeanah [35] found that 50% of a sample of 3- to 6-year-old children met criteria for PTSD. To put this in perspective, in a study of nonreferred preschool children recruited from pediatric clinics in North Carolina [39], only 0.6% of children met criteria for PTSD.

Second, in keeping with previous research, the degree of exposure to hurricane-related events seems to be related to the degree of symptomatology later [34,35,37]. Scheeringa and Zeanah [35] dichotomized their sample into those who evacuated before the hurricane and those who remained in the city. Not surprisingly, more of the group that stayed (34% of the total sample) met diagnostic criteria for PTSD, but more than 40% of those who evacuated before the storm (66% of the total sample) also met criteria for PTSD. The traumatic event cited by most of the evacuated group was returning to their damaged or destroyed homes. This surprising finding was not accounted for by increased vulnerability, because there was no difference in pre-Katrina levels of symptomatology, at least as reported retrospectively by parents.

Third, moderators of the effects of the hurricane on children's symptomatology remain either unexplored or unclear. One important vulnerability factor increasing risk for PTSD symptoms was anxiety before the storm [37]. Surprisingly, neither ethnicity nor gender emerged as important moderators. This finding may indicate either that ethnicity and gender were not important moderators or that the studies were limited by sample sizes and narrow ranges of children. Although Osofsky and colleagues [8] reported that 37% of the children in their survey reported previous trauma or loss, Scheeringa and Zeanah [35] found the number of prior adverse events did not affect symptomatology after Katrina. This area deserves more work. Also, in the 2007 survey by Osofsky and colleagues [8], parents reported higher levels of symptoms among young children who had been separated from caregivers during the hurricane and its aftermath. On the other hand, Scheeringa and Zeanah [35] found no differences in PTSD symptomatology or diagnoses in preschool children who were or were not separated during the evacuation (20% of the sample) or experienced displacement (37% of the sample). Perhaps the children studied had maintained contact with at least one important caregiver despite separation from a parent, and this contact may have buffered the effects. In any case, this issue also deserves more attention.

Fourth, it is well established that approximately 80% to 90% of individuals who have PTSD have at least one comorbid psychiatric disorder [40]. In the group of preschool children studied by Scheeringa and Zeanah [35], PTSD was comorbid with at least one other disorder 88.6% of the time. Furthermore, the onset of new disorders was always accompanied by PTSD symptomatology. This finding provides cross-age replication of the finding that traumatic events that cause PTSD also lead to a host of other behavioral problems that need individualized clinical attention. Further research is needed on how best to understand and treat these comorbid clusters of disorders.

Fifth, although only two intervention studies in children have been completed to date, both report positive effects on trauma symptoms. Weems and colleagues [31] designed and implemented an intervention comprising relaxation training combined with hierarchical exposures. Results indicated that the intervention reduced test anxiety symptoms, was related to relative academic improvement and reduced posttraumatic symptoms in ninth grade students. Salloum and Overstreet [38] evaluated a manualized 10-week-long intervention that employed cognitive behavioral and narrative therapy strategies. A total of 56 school-aged children who had moderate-to-severe posttraumatic symptoms were assigned randomly to individual or group intervention in January 2006. The intervention effectively and significantly reduced symptoms of posttraumatic stress, depression, and traumatic grief in children following Hurricane Katrina. There were no differences between individual or group administration of the intervention.

These intervention studies emphasize that evidence-based treatments for PTSD in children are available and feasible and that it is important to implement them sooner rather than later in a postdisaster environment. The lack of availability of such treatments for all the children and adolescents who could benefit from them has been one of the most unfortunate characteristics of the post-Katrina mental health response.

Limitations of research to date

Obviously, these studies of the effects of Hurricane Katrina on children's mental health are early reports with significant limitations. All are limited by their cross-sectional designs; some are limited by reliance on measures of limited validity, and others are limited by the use of single-informant, self-report methods. An important limitation affecting almost all of the studies is sampling. This limitation is necessarily the result of more than 150,000 residents still being displaced. It is reasonable to assume that many of the most affected are not available for research being conducted in the city. If anything, the dramatic findings regarding children's outcomes are likely to be understated rather than overstated.

Lessons learned

Clinical issues

As with many issues that were illuminated by the Hurricane Katrina disaster, the gap between what was and is known about the need for treatment and intervention and what actually was provided is unacceptably large. PTSD has been a well-researched phenomena since it was described formally in 1980 [41], with an enormous number of studies addressing assessment, longitudinal course, concomitant disability, and effective treatments, including high-quality research in children and adolescents.

It has been well known that PTSD develops immediately after traumatic events, including disasters. In one study, PTSD developed within the first month in 98% of cases [42]. Nearly all individuals who are exposed to life-threatening events develop some symptomatology of PTSD right away, but only about 30% have enduring symptomatology beyond 1 month [40]. Therefore, any delay in providing treatment after 1 month is contraindicated, and any planned efforts to "wait for PTSD to develop" beyond this window would be remarkably uninformed by modern research.

It has been well known that for individuals whose symptoms persist beyond a month, PTSD tends to be chronic. Rates of PTSD after 1 year were 47% in one large study [42], and symptoms persisted for more than 3 years in one third of subjects in another large study [43]. The findings in children are similar, if not worse. In a study of children affected by Hurricane Andrew, 53% had no change in PTSD symptoms 21 months after the event, and PTSD symptoms actually worsened in 17% [44]. Older children exposed to a bushfire in Australia showed no improvement in PTSD symptomatology after 18 months [45]. Even traumatized preschool children showed no decrease in PTSD symptoms over 2 years [46]. The obvious clinical implication is that after the early weeks or months, symptoms do not improve naturally, and treatment is required.

It has been well known that exposure-based therapies, such as cognitive behavioral therapy and prolonged exposure therapy, are effective for most individuals who have PTSD, including children [47]. Other treatments that have shown effectiveness mostly in adult studies, such as eye-movement desensitization and reprocessing therapy [48] and pharmacotherapy with selective serotonin reuptake agonists [49], can be applied in informed fashions to children and adolescents.

Policy issues

The scale of the Hurricane Katrina disaster made it clear that governmental and private community plans for postdisaster psychiatric needs were not sufficient, and the low priority given to psychiatric needs in the recovery period has ensured that mental health recovery is slow. Even in major but relatively lesser future disasters, when only sectors of a city are incapacitated and neighboring sectors still can function to pick up the slack, it is unlikely that most communities will have enough clinicians trained in techniques of evidence-based treatment for children and adolescents who have PTSD. Because it is not feasible for outside clinicians to work for months in distant locations to provide full courses of therapy, there must be a greater commitment to support and train local clinicians who are willing to do this work after disasters. Evidence-based treatment for trauma following disasters needs to be implemented on a large-scale basis in the initial period following a disaster. Rapid funding to support training in evidence-based treatments is needed, and because of the substantial initial financial commitment, the scale of such an effort would require support by the federal government.

This need is well beyond the federal government's current commitment to fund crisis counseling, which is a well-intentioned program but is not treatment and is unproven even for its meager aims of facilitating referrals to actual treatment. FEMA and SAMHSA need to develop guidelines that permit and encourage actual treatment among the services they provide. Doing so may require amending or reinterpreting the Stafford Act.

Furthermore, the current guidelines are too restrictive in allowing only state agencies to receive federal disaster funding. Broadening the pool of eligible recipients beyond traditionally nonprogressive and administratively top-heavy state agencies will increase competition for high-quality programs and provide alternatives to the single point-of-entry through a state agency. Federal-to-local partnerships, such as those for Head Start programs, might be a more flexible model to explore. Allowing local agencies to receive federal mental health funding also might channel funds to relatively more functional and indigenous managers and staff for these short-term projects.

Last, every program, whether CCP or treatment, should have a high-quality program evaluation component to begin the effort to determine if the goals of the program are being met and resources (eg, taxpayer dollars) are used wisely. As noted earlier, the CCP programs that are funded with millions of dollars every year in this country require anonymous contacts with individuals, making accountability a de facto impossibility. A congressional oversight agency has recommended twice that FEMA and SAMHSA evaluate the CCP program, and this recommendation has been ignored twice. Real strengthening of the program requires, at a minimum, eliminating the anonymity rule, accepting the use of standardized measures, encouraging state-of-the-art interventions that are supported by evidence, and conducting follow-up assessments.

Although the relationship between disasters and trauma in children and adolescents is widely recognized, facts that are well known among researchers do not seem to be fully appreciated by those allocating federal funding for postdisaster clinical responses. An adequate and modern mental health response in the future will require a timely, well-staffed, adequately funded, accountable, and well-managed plan for actual treatment. This response would require a level of funding that can be furnished only by the federal government. If this policy could emerge from the havoc wrought by Katrina, it would provide some meaning for those who suffered so much and some hope for future victims.

References

[1] Canino G, Bravo M, Rubio-Stipec M. The impact of disaster on mental health: prospective and retrospective analyses. Int J Ment Health 1990;19(1):51–69.

[2] Satcher D, Friel S, Bell R. Natural and manmade disasters and mental health. JAMA 2007; 298(12):2540–2.

[3] Dalton R, Scheeringa M, Zeanah C. Did the prevalence of PTSD following Hurricane Katrina match a rapid needs assessment prediction? A template for future public planning after large-scale disasters. Psychiatric Annals 2008;38:134–41.

[4] Brodie M, Weltzien E, Altman D, et al. Experiences of Hurricane Katrina evacuees in Houston shelters: implications for future planning. Am J Public Health 2006;96(8): 1402–8.

[5] Federal Emergency Management Agency. Hurricane Katrina. Available at: http://www. fema.gov/pdf/hazard/hurricane/2005katrina/locations_applicants_combined_map.pdf. Accessed October 25, 2007.

[6] Hunter M. Schools take in displaced students. Available at: CNN.com. Accessed October 26, 2007.

[7] National Center for Missing and Exploited Children. National center for missing and exploited children reunites last missing child separated by Hurricane Katrina and Rita. After six months, all missing/displaced children are back home with their families. Alexandria (VA): National Center for Missing and Exploited Children; March 17, 2006.

[8] Osofsky J, Osofsky H, Harris W. Katrina's children: social policy considerations for children in disasters. Soc Policy Rep 2007;21:3–18.

[9] Mittal A. History of the Lake Pontchartrain and Vicinity Hurricane Protection Project: GAO-06-244T. United States Government Accountability Office. Available at: www.gao. gov/new.items/d06244t.pdf. Accessed October 20, 2007.

[10] Rudowitz R, Rowland D, Shartzer A. Health care in New Orleans before and after Hurricane Katrina. Health Aff 2006;25(5):393–406.

[11] Brown A. Hurricane Katrina pummels three states. Transcript of CNN Newsnight with Aaron Brown. August 29, 2006.

[12] Rulon M, Scott K. Evacuation plan failed to consider those without transportation. Burlington Free Press. March 11, 2006. Available at: http://www.burlingtonfreepress.com/apps/ pbcs.dll/article?AID=/20050905/NEWS01/509050309/1009. Accessed July, 2007.

[13] Associated Press. Storm's victims unlike most Americans: census analysis shows how demographics of poverty contributed to disaster. Available at: msnbc.com. Accessed October 30, 2007.

[14] Webster R. Teen mental health care center in N.O. is in limbo. New Orleans City Business. May 15, 2006. Available at: http://www.neworleanscitybusiness.com/viewFeature.cfm? recID=390.

[15] McConnaughty J. Charity system opens new psych hospital. Leesville Daily Leader. September 25, 2007.

[16] Maggi L, Moran K. Mental patients have nowhere to go. The Times-Picayune. April 22, 2007. p. 4.

[17] Moran K. Psychiatric hospital to open uptown, LSU to run center on DePaul campus. The Times-Picayune. February 14, 2007:A1. p. 1.

[18] Wang P, Gruber M, Powers R, et al. Disruption of existing mental health treatments and failure to initiate new treatment after Hurricane Katrina. Am J Psychiatry 2008;165:34–41.

[19] Robert T. Stafford Disaster Relief and Emergency Assistance Act. Pub. L 106-390, § 1(a), 114 Stat. 1552.

[20] Sundararaman R, Lister S, Williams E. Gulf Coast hurricanes: addressing survivors' mental health and substance abuse treatment needs. The Library of Congress; November 29, 2006. RL33738. Available at: www.nyrag.org/usr_doc/CRSKatrina.pdf. Accessed September 28, 2007.

[21] Zeanah C, Larrieu J, Heller S, et al. Evaluation of a preventive intervention for maltreated infants and toddlers in foster care. J Am Acad Child Adolesc Psychiatry 2001;40:214–21.

[22] Gritter K. Program addresses students' mental health—behavior Times-Picayune, section Metairie. October 1, 2006. p. 1.

[23] Available at: www.wkkf.org. Accessed December 21, 2007.

[24] Available at: www.project-fleur-de-lis.org. Accessed December 21, 2007.

[25] Adelman H, Taylor L. Safe schools in the context of school improvement. Paper presented at the 2007 National Conference on Safe Schools, 2007; Hamilton Fish Institute, Washington, DC: July 9–15, 2005.

[26] Drell M. NOAH update. The Louisiana Psychiatric Medical Association Newsletter 2007; 42(4):6–7.

[27] Conrad E, Townsend M, Buccola N. Restoration of mental health services in New Orleans. Am J Psychiatry 2008;165:33.

[28] Abramson D, Garfield R. The recovery divide: poverty and the widening gap among Mississippi children and families affected by Hurricane Katrina. New York: Mississippi Child & Family Health Study, National Center for Disaster Preparedness, The Children's Health Fund; 2007.

[29] Assessment of health-related needs after Hurricanes Katrina and Rita: Orleans and Jefferson Parishes, New Orleans area, Louisiana, October 17–22, 2005. MMWR Morb Mortal Wkly Rep 2006. p. 38–41.

[30] Abramson D, Garfield R. On the edge: children and families displaced by Hurricanes Katrina and Rita face a looming medical and mental health crisis. National Center or Disaster Preparedness, Operation Assist. Available at: www.ncdp.mailman.columbia.edu/program_special.htm. Accessed July 9, 2006.

[31] Weisler R, Barbee J, Townsend M. Mental health and recovery in the Gulf Coast after Hurricanes Katrina and Rita. JAMA 2006;296(5):585–8.

[32] Nossiter A. After the storm, students left alone and angry. The New York Times, front page. November 1, 2006.

[33] Weems CF, Taylor LK, Marks AB, et al. The impact of hurricane Katrina on disadvantaged adolescents: A prospective study with results of a school based intervention. Meeting of the Society for Research on Adolescence, Chicago, IL. March 6–9, 2008.

[34] Hensley L, Varela R. PTSD symptoms and somatic complaints following Hurricane Katrina: the role of trait anxiety and anxiety sensitivity. J Clin Child Adolesc Psychol, in press.

[35] Scheeringa M, Zeanah C. Reconsideration of harm's way: onsets and comorbidity patterns in preschool children and their caregivers following Hurricane Katrina. J Clin Child Adolesc Psychol, in press.

[36] Scaramella L. A test of the Family Stress Model on toddler-aged children's adjustment among Hurricane Katrina impacted and non-impacted low income families. J Clin Child Adolesc Psychol, in press.

[37] Weems C, Pina A, Costa N, et al. Predisaster trait anxiety and negative affect predict posttraumatic stress in youths after Hurricane Katrina. J Consult Clin Psychol 2007;75(1): 154–9.

[38] Salloum A, Overstreet S. Effectiveness of a grief and trauma intervention for children post disaster. J Clin Child Adolesc Psychol, in press.

[39] Egger H, Erkanli A, Keeler G, et al. Test-retest reliability of the Preschool Age Psychiatric Assessment (PAPA). J Am Acad Child Adolesc Psychiatry 2006;45:538–49.

[40] Kessler R, Sonnega A, Bromet E, et al. Posttraumatic stress disorder in the National Comorbidity Survey. Arch Gen Psychiatry 1995;52:1048–60.

[41] American Psychiatric Association. Diagnostic and statistical manual. 3rd edition. Washington, DC: American Psychiatric Association; 1980. p. 236–8.

[42] Davidson J, Hughes G, Blazer D, et al. Posttraumatic stress disorder in the community: an epidemiologic study. Psychol Med 1991;21:713–21.

[43] Helzer J, Robins L, McEvoy M. Post-traumatic stress disorder in the general population. N Engl J Med 1987;317:1630–4.

[44] Shaw J, Applegate B, Schorr C. Twenty-one-month follow-up study of school-age children exposed to Hurricane Andrew. J Am Acad Child Adolesc Psychiatry 1995;35(3):359–64.

[45] McFarlane A. Posttraumatic phenomena in a longitudinal study of children following a natural disaster. J Am Acad Child Adolesc Psychiatry 1987;26:764–9.

[46] Scheeringa M, Zeanah C, Myers L, et al. Predictive validity in a prospective follow-up of PTSD in preschool children. J Am Acad Child Adolesc Psychiatry 2005;44(9):899–906.

[47] Cohen J, Deblinger E, Mannarino A, et al. A multisite, randomized controlled trial for children with sexual abuse-related PTSD symptoms. J Am Acad Child Adolesc Psychiatry 2004;43(4):393–402.

[48] Bradley R, Greene J, Russ E, et al. A multidimensional meta-analysis of psychotherapy for PTSD. Am J Psychiatry 2005;162:214–27.

[49] Schoenfeld F, Marmar C, Neylan T. Current concepts in pharmacotherapy of posttraumatic stress disorder. Psychiatr Serv 2004;55(5):519–31.

ELSEVIER
SAUNDERS

Child Adolesc Psychiatric Clin N Am
17 (2008) 703–712

CHILD AND
ADOLESCENT
PSYCHIATRIC CLINICS
OF NORTH AMERICA

Index

Note: Page numbers of article titles are in **boldface** type.

1056-4993/08/$ - see front matter © 2008 Elsevier Inc. All rights reserved.
doi:10.1016/S1056-4993(08)00035-7   *childpsych.theclinics.com*